Scintimammography
A guide to good practice

This book has been developed to assist nuclear medicine physicians and technologists in undertaking scintimammography of women with suspected or proven breast cancer. Additionally, it reviews the value of scintimammography, particularly with ^{99m}Tc sestamibi, in diagnosis, evaluation and development of management strategies. Therefore, we hope that it will provide an introduction to the potential benefits of scintimammography for oncologists, surgeons and radiotherapists.

The authors wish to acknowledge the contribution of Ms Gail Lowe in the preparation of the manuscript and of Du Pont Pharma Radiopharmaceuticals who provided an educational grant.

John Buscombe, MBBS, MSc, MD, FRCP
Consultant in Nuclear Medicine
Department of Nuclear Medicine, Royal Free Hospital and
School of Medicine, London, UK

Jonathan Hill, MB ChB, DMRD, FRCR
Consultant Radiologist, Nuclear Medicine
Preston Acute Hospital NHS Trust, Preston, UK

Santilal Parbhoo, MB ChB, PhD, FRCS
Consultant Surgeon, Breast Unit
University Department of Surgery, Royal Free Hospital and
School of Medicine, London, UK

Publisher

Gibbs Associates Limited, Edgbaston House,
3 Duchess Place, Edgbaston, Birmingham B16 8NH, England.

British Library Cataloguing in Publication Data

A catalogue record for this book is available from the British Library.
ISBN 1 902018 01 X

Printed and bound in Great Britain by The Alternative Design & Printing Company,
Birmingham.

Front cover: Lateral sestamibi scintimammography showing focal uptake in breast cancer

Contents

Chapter One

Introduction

Introduction

Incidence of breast cancer

The incidence of breast cancer has increased steadily in most European countries over the last 40 years. It is now the most common malignancy in women in Europe, Australasia, North America and much of Latin America.[1] (Figure 1) In these countries recent figures suggest that women have a life-time risk of developing the disease of 1 in 12, although in some societies the rate rises to 1 in 8.[3,4] By the year 2000, the number of new cases diagnosed annually is predicted to be 1.1-1.4 million.[5]

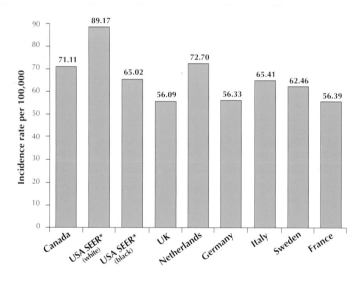

* SEER = Surveillance, epidemiology and end results program

Figure 1   Incidence of new cases of breast cancer per 100,000 women in Europe and North America (age - standardised to world population, 1983-1987) [2]

Mortality from breast cancer

In many Western countries, breast cancer is the leading cause of death in women aged 35-54. The actual mortality figures vary from country to country but range between 1.5-4%.[2] (Figure 2) Despite the increased incidence, mortality has remained relatively stable. This has been attributed to i) an improvement in breast cancer treatment; ii) more cases of breast cancer being diagnosed due to screening; iii) identification of non-fatal cancers; and, iv) a combination of these three reasons.[5,6]

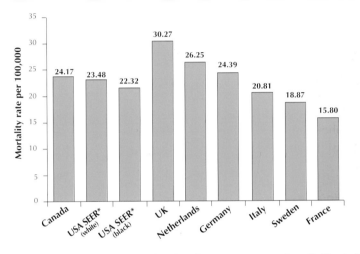

* SEER = Surveillance, epidemiology and end results program   From Parkin *et al* 1992

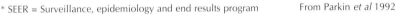

Figure 2   Mortality from breast cancer per 100,000 women in Europe and North America (age - standardised to world population, 1983-1987) [2]

Risk factors for breast cancer

Risk factors for developing breast cancer have been identified[5] of which increasing age is the most important as a woman aged >50 years presenting with a breast lump is five times more likely to have breast cancer than a woman <50 years.[7]

Established

- Age
- Demographic characteristics
- Previous breast cancer
- Carcinoma *in situ*
- Benign breast disease
- Family history
- Genetic predisposition
- Hormone replacement therapy
- Irradiation of the breast
- Factors related to menses
  - early menarche and late menopause
- Factors related to pregnancy
- Mammographic parenchymal pattern
- Obesity
- Oral contraceptives

Possible

- Alcohol
- Breast feeding
- Diet
- Physical activity

The role of screening programmes

Early detection and correct diagnosis will determine the final prognosis of a patient with breast cancer. If tumours are detected when they are small and localised, the clinical outcome is likely to be better. Therefore, in many countries, screening programmes have been introduced generally employing mammography. Mammography provides effective early diagnosis and has been shown to save lives. (Table 1) Randomised controlled trials demonstrate a 17% reduction in mortality for women entering mammographic screening programmes between the ages of 40 and 49 years. Some studies show a 25-30% reduction for patients over 50 years.[8-11]

- Cost effective technique for screening large populations
- Identifies breast cancer at early stages of the disease
- Sensitive technique
- Reduces mortality

Table 1   The benefits of mammographic screening

4

Limitations of mammographic screening programmes

Screening programmes are designed to test for initial signs of breast cancer in large numbers of the population. Therefore, they need to be cost effective and provide an acceptable sensitivity. Mammography fulfils these criteria, although its limitations with respect to sensitivity and specificity have been demonstrated when used as a diagnostic tool.[12] As a result, mammography is usually the first diagnostic step. Follow-up tests are required to confirm the exact nature of a lesion seen on a screening mammogram.

KEY POINTS

- In Western countries, breast cancer is the most common cancer in women
- It is the major cause of death in women under the age of 50 years
- Screening for breast cancer, early correct diagnosis and prompt effective treatment reduce mortality
- Mammography is the most commonly used screening modality
- Further tests are required to confirm mammographic findings

Chapter Two

The diagnosis of breast cancer

The diagnosis of breast cancer

Suspected breast cancer may be identified by a screening mammogram. However, media attention and improved health education have increased women's awareness about breast cancer, particularly the value of early detection by self-examination. Therefore, many women present to their physicians as a result of finding a suspicious lump on self-examination. Irrespective of whether a patient presents as a result of self-examination or referral from a screening programme, many questions need to be answered. The nature, size and malignancy of the abnormality must be evaluated once the diagnosis is confirmed and a treatment plan developed. Therefore, the diagnosis of breast cancer is based on information gathered from a number of sources including the patient's history, a clinical examination, medical imaging and biopsy. (Table 1)

● Medical history
● Clinical examination (inspection and palpation)
● Medical imaging (mammography, ultrasonography, scintimammography)
● Biopsy

Table 1   Data used in the diagnosis of breast cancer

Following a physical examination, imaging provides further diagnostic information. A pathological diagnosis can only be made after examining tissue obtained from either a fine needle aspiration biopsy (FNAB) or a core biopsy (CB). However, some biopsies may only be possible in combination with imaging techniques. For example, ultrasound is used to guide a biopsy on a mammographically identified abnormality which is impalpable.

In some developed countries, about 1 in 4 women undergo a surgical biopsy because of a suspicious breast lesion.[1] In North America, where this is commonly done, the majority of these women will not have cancer. As a result, unnecessary biopsies cause anxiety and stress for women which may be reduced if imaging techniques can more accurately differentiate malignant from benign masses. A complication can arise if scars from biopsies cause future mammograms to be read as abnormal. This can mean some women undergo several biopsies, all of which are negative.

Several currently available imaging techniques provide further diagnostic information. These include "spot" mammography, high density ultrasonography, magnetic resonance imaging (MRI), computed tomography (CT), nuclear medicine techniques and positron emission tomography (PET). Each of these techniques has advantages and disadvantages.

Scintimammography, using either planar or single photon emission computed tomography (SPECT), is a new nuclear imaging technique in breast cancer used to confirm the presence or absence of breast cancer.

Imaging techniques for the diagnosis of breast cancer

Mammography
Mammography is an X-ray of the breast which can pinpoint abnormalities. To obtain clear, precise images for accurate diagnosis, the breast is compressed firmly for the short duration of the X-ray requiring a low dose of radiation. Two views are performed: i) cranio-candal and ii) lateral oblique. The result is a grey-scale image of the architecture of the breast which needs to be interpreted by a radiologist or physician.

Aberrations are identified by comparing patterns of density differences. Areas of density such as calcifications and dense glandular tissue appear as white, whilst fatty tissue presents as black. Abnormalities are normally focal areas of dense tissue containing specks of calcium. These spiculated areas show up as specific white patterns. Calcifications and dense glandular breast tissue also appear white on a mammogram making it difficult to differentiate cancers from other structural abnormalities. (Figure 1)

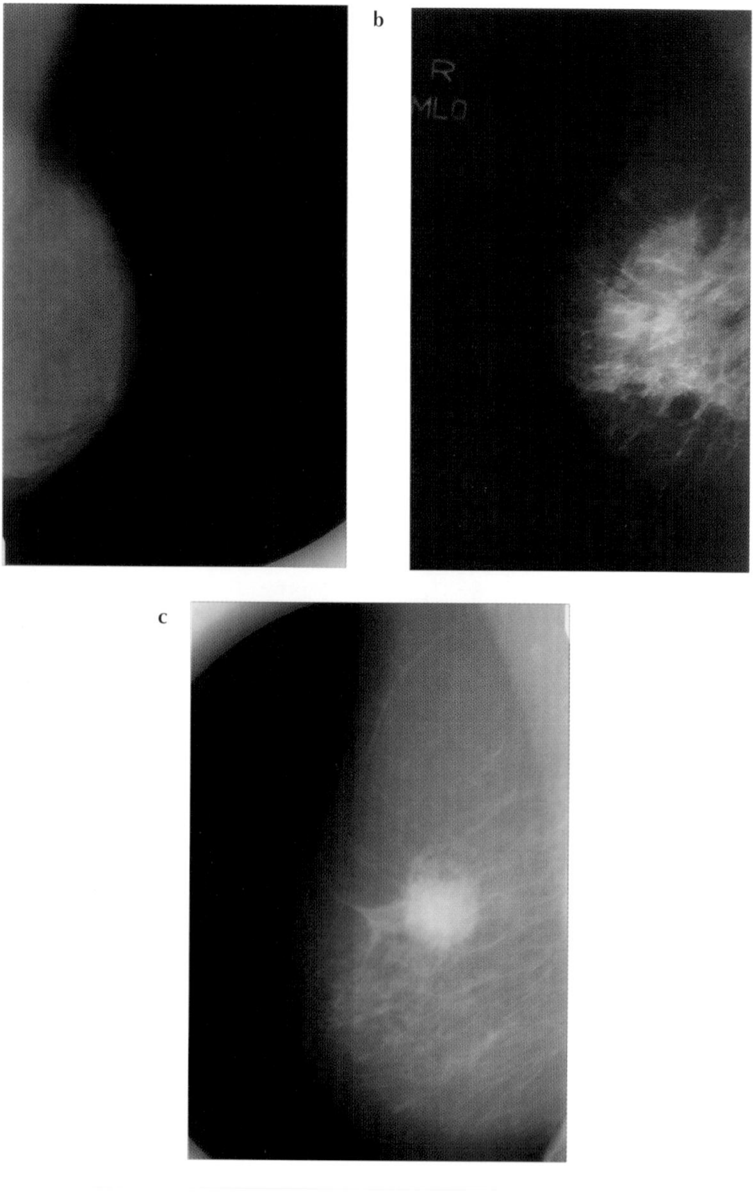

Figure 1   Mammographic images showing (a) dense tissue, (b) calcification and (c) cancer

Other factors may complicate the mammographic diagnosis of breast cancer. For example, patients who have undergone previous breast surgery may have scars which appear similar to cancerous lesions on a mammogram. Meanwhile, radiation therapy can thicken breast tissue and breast implants can mask the presence of a cancer. (Figure 2)

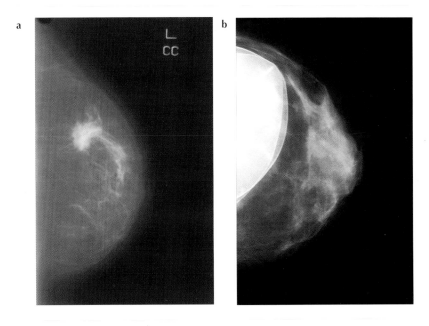

Figure 2   Mammographic images of (a) scarred breast tissue and (b) implant

Mammography can identify areas of increased density which are not entirely characteristic of cancer or benign disease. Thus, the mammogram is *non-diagnostic* or *equivocal*. (Table 2) Where mammograms are read by two radiologists, the number of equivocal mammograms can be reduced. However, about 10% of diagnostic mammograms may still be reported as equivocal[2] and further evaluation using an additional technique is needed to obtain a diagnosis.

The false-positive rate for mammography is high because many benign lesions result in calcifications which may be reported as suspicious.

- Dense glandular breasts
- Glandular lumpy breasts with diffuse areas of increased and decreased density
- Fibrocystic breasts where it may be difficult to determine the exact reason for highlighted abnormalities
- Previous breast surgery
- Non-spiculated calcifications in the breast
- Multi-focal or multi-centric lesions where the extent of cancer may be underestimated
- Breast implants

Table 2   Factors resulting in non-diagnostic or equivocal mammograms

Sensitivities of between 63-90% have been reported[3] and depend on various factors including the quality of the image and the experience of the reader. The low specificity of mammography often leads to excisional biopsy for benign breast changes.

The positive predictive rate of mammography (the probability that a positive test is positive for cancer) varies, but a range of 10-50% has been reported.[4] This suggests that although mammography is highly effective as a screening modality, there are patients in whom it is non-diagnostic. Therefore, other imaging techniques are necessary to increase diagnostic certainty.

Ultrasound imaging

Ultrasound imaging employs sound waves which are reflected from different tissue structures to create an image. For example, the most common cause of breast mass in perimenopausal women is a cyst or cystic changes within the breast. The echogenic pattern of such fluid-filled spaces is very different to that produced by solid lesions such as tumours. (Figure 3) Therefore, ultrasound complements screening mammography and palpation.

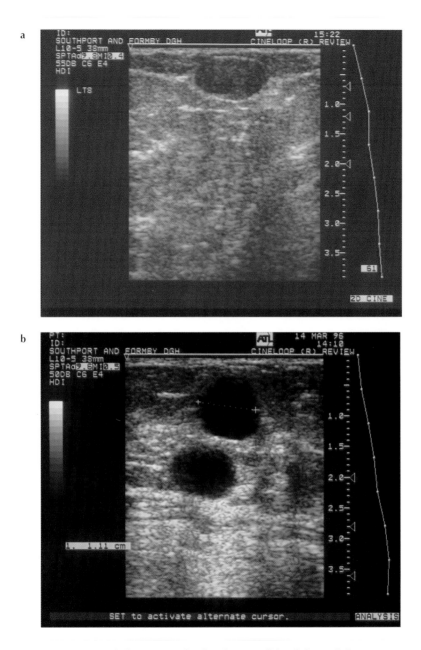

Figure 3   Images of ultrasonography showing (a) solid and (b) cystic breast tumours

The sensitivity of ultrasound for small lesions is low, although modern ultrasonography using a 7.5-10 MHz probe has detected small, clinically occult carcinomas. The same studies reported a corresponding 25% reduction in unnecessary excisional biopsies compared to using mammography alone.[5,6] However, ultrasound with the standard breast probes does not detect microcalcifications, nor can it detect very small tumours. High density ultrasound imaging with a 13 MHz probe allows detection of areas of microcalcification.

Therefore, ultrasound imaging answers many questions about palpable lesions but its specificity depends on where the location of the lesion is in the breast, the quality of the machine and the expertise of the technician. Results may be improved when Doppler flow studies are used, although further research is required. Optimally, ultrasound is used in young women with full glandular breasts because of their intrinsic density on mammography. Ultrasound allows rapid assessment of a palpable lump as to whether it is solid or cystic. It is also used by surgeons as a guide when performing biopsies.[7]

Magnetic resonance imaging

Magnetic resonance imaging (MRI) produces excellent three-dimensional images of breast structure. (Figure 4) It has a high sensitivity (86-100%) and identifies lesions of only 2-3mm. Multi-centric disease with no microcalcifications has also been diagnosed.[8] However, MRI has a relatively low specificity (27-97%)[9] and many centres reported specificities of <40% in the detection of primary breast cancer. Therefore, further research is needed to improve this technique.[10,11,12]

To obtain good magnetic resonance images, the breast must be placed within a special coil to ensure a high magnetic field within the breast. Different sequences can be used to image patients including high resolution, rapid imaging, dynamic imaging and fat suppression. The most popular are the fat suppression T_2 weighted sequences while dynamic imaging has provided the highest specificity to-date.[7] An advantage of MRI is that it identifies both benign and malignant lesions because of their differing temporal and morphologic patterns of contrast enhancement.[8]

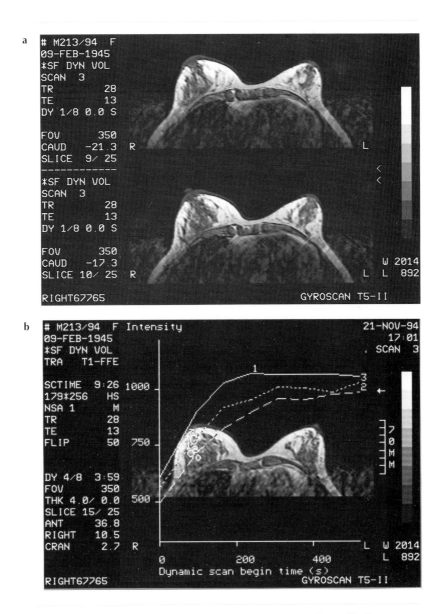

*Figure 4   MRI breast image showing examples of contrast enhanced lesions
(a) pre-enhancement and (b) contrast enhanced curve*

Research to improve the specificity of MRI by using gadolinium uptake and wash-out rates has proved promising. Gadolinium-DTPA enhanced MRI can distinguish post-operative radiation scarring from tumour recurrence.[13] The specificity of MRI can be marginally improved by analysing Gd-DTPA kinetics which can also provide important information about the heterogeneity, permeability and vascularity of lesions.[14]

Nuclear medicine imaging techniques

Nuclear medicine imaging techniques depend on the physiological distribution of a radiolabelled tracer. This tracer (a radionuclide) is normally attached to a carrier molecule (a metabolite) and together they form a radiopharmaceutical. In most cases, this is injected into a peripheral vein and circulates around the body.

Cancer cells are hungry for metabolites such as glucose and, therefore, take up the metabolite along with any associated radiotracer. Because cancer cells are more metabolically active than the cells surrounding them, a concentration of the radiotracer builds up in the cancer cell. (Figure 5) This appears as an area of increased focal uptake when imaged with a gamma camera.

Examples of radiotracers include fluorinated glucose used in positron emission tomography and thallium-201 (a potassium analogue) which can be used with a standard nuclear medicine camera. Other nuclear medicine techniques might use the increased vascularity of a tumour, or local tissue oedema caused by the tumour, to identify a cancer.

It may also be possible to use antibodies labelled with a radiotracer such as the epidermal growth factor receptor or the oestrogen receptor. Again, the aim is to have more radiotracer at the site of the cancer than in the surrounding tissue. The cancer then appears as an obvious area of increased activity. A more direct method would be to use a radio-labelled receptor agonist such as indium-111 octreotide. This could

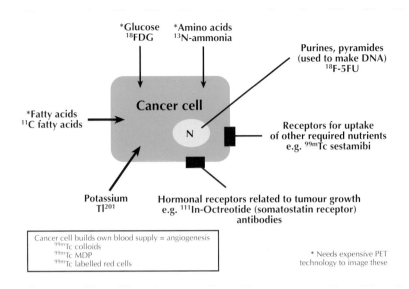

Figure 5 Cell and metabolites

locate somatostatin receptors on cancer cells which occur in about 30% of breast cancers. (Figure 6) However, none of these agents have undergone formal trials or have been evaluated for diagnosing breast cancer to-date.

A further nuclear medicine technique used in breast cancer does not image the breast directly but identifies the sentinel node in the lymph nodes draining a particular cancer. Identifying the sentinel node is important in staging breast cancer. A small amount of radiolabelled colloid is injected into the tissue above the cancer. This is followed through the lymph channels by imaging and using a hand held intra-operative probe.

Positron emission tomography (PET)

Positron emission tomography (PET) uses positron/electron alienation patterns to study metabolic reactions in body systems. It is proving promising for differentiating benign from malignant breast masses, determining how far a cancer has progressed and predicting patient

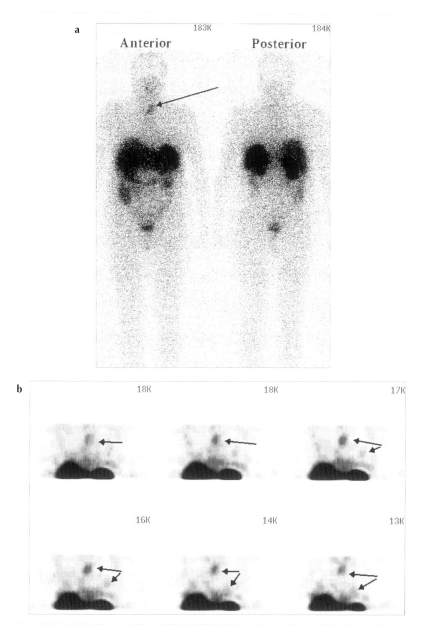

Figure 6   (a) whole body and (b) chest SPECT images of indium -111 octreotide image showing somatostatin receptor in metastatic breast cancer

survival after the cancer is removed. However, its expense and limited availability rule it out as a routine modality for clinical diagnosis.

Nevertheless, [18]FDG PET can distinguish benign from malignant primary breast lesions with a sensitivity of 96% and specificity of 100%.[15,16,17] Metastases in the axilla have also been assessed with a sensitivity of 90% and specificity of 100%.[17] This area is difficult to accurately image using many other imaging techniques.

Among the main advantages PET imaging has over mammography and ultrasound is that it can provide functional information *in vivo*. Information on the metabolic activity, vascularisation, oxygen consumption and the tumour's receptor status can be obtained.[18] Such information is useful in characterising tumours and assessing prognosis. However, PET's role may be in determining the presence of recurrent breast cancer.

Scintimammography using planar and SPECT imaging

Scintimammography is a nuclear imaging technique which can deliver breast imaging as sensitive as X-ray mammography and MRI in palpable tumours but with greater specificity.[19] (Figure 7) The data obtained can significantly increase the understanding of the nature of any breast lesions. It also provides complementary images for the diagnosis and treatment of breast cancer.

A variety of radiopharmaceuticals have been investigated in breast cancer with varying degrees of success. They are discussed fully in the following chapter. However, methoxyisobutylisonitrile (sestamibi) has proved to be the most valuable for the evaluation of patients with non-diagnostic mammograms. Sensitivities of 86-95% have been reported in sestamibi studies for palpable breast tumours and 60-91% in non-palpable tumours.[19] Specificity values have been 62-93%.[19] Further explanation and discussion of scintimammography using both planar and SPECT imaging appears in the following chapters.

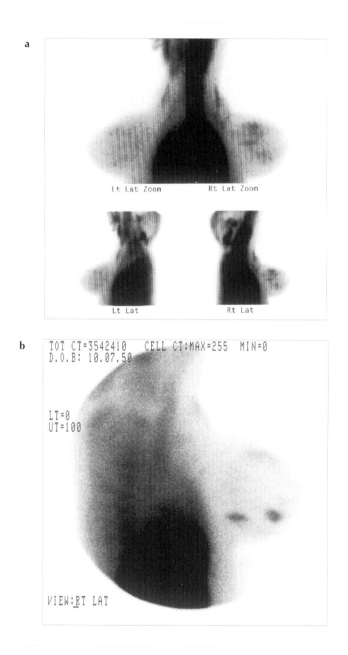

Figure 7   Scintimammogram showing (a) multi-centric and (b) multi-focal cancers

	Strengths	Weaknesses
Mammography	● Relatively inexpensive ● Widely available ● Architectural image ● High sensitivity	● Low specificity ● About 10% of structures are equivocal ● Non-diagnostic in patients with dense breasts, implants and scarring ● Not all patients can tolerate breast compression
Ultrasound	● Relatively inexpensive ● Widely available ● Architectural image ● Used to differentiate benign from malignant lesions ● Provides a biopsy guide	● Low sensitivity ● Specificity dependent on location of lesion and expertise of technician
MRI	● High sensitivity ● Architectural image ● Can differentiate between benign and malignant lesions	● Relatively expensive ● Not widely available ● Low specificity
PET	● Can differentiate between benign and malignant lesions ● High sensitivity ● High specificity ● Can image axilla	● Expensive ● Not widely available
Scintimammography	● Relatively inexpensive ● Widely available ● High sensitivity in palpable lesions ● High specificity ● Functional imaging ● Can image axilla ● Can provide planar and SPECT images	● Low sensitivity in lesions <1cm

Imaging techniques used in the diagnosis of breast cancer: Strengths and weaknesses

KEY POINTS

- The diagnosis of breast cancer is best made using a multi-modality strategy
- Unnecessary biopsies cause distress and anxiety to patients which may be reduced if less invasive diagnostic procedures provide effective diagnosis
- Mammography is a sensitive technique although specificity is low
- Mammography in certain groups of women produces images which are difficult to interpret, requiring further investigations
- Ultrasonography can provide important information about the nature of solid or cystic breast lumps although sensitivity is low in small lesions
- MRI produces high quality anatomical images of the breast with a sensitivity approaching 100% but with a very low specificity
- PET images are highly sensitive and specific although the technique is expensive and only available in certain specialist centres
- Scintimammography provides comparable sensitivity to mammography with higher specificity

The authors wish to acknowledge Dr Anita Brown, Consultant Radiologist from Southport and District General Hospital for supplying images for use within this chapter

Chapter Three

The rationale for scintimammography

The rationale for scintimammography

Nuclear medicine is a well established imaging modality in many areas of medicine. Today, scintimammography is one of the most promising new areas for nuclear medicine providing referring surgeons and oncologists with valuable data in diagnosis and treatment.

Scintimammography requires the intravenous administration of a suitable radiotracer followed by the acquisition of an emission image using a gamma camera to identify the presence and site of a lesion. This noninvasive procedure provides functional and biological information (Figure 1) complementing other anatomical imaging produced by mammography, ultrasonography or MRI.[1]

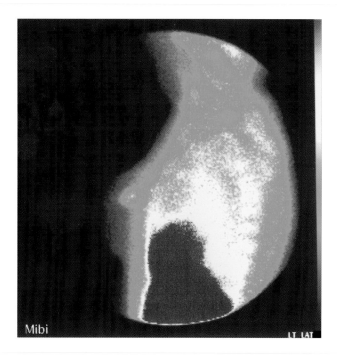

Figure 1 ^{99m}Tc sestamibi scintimammogram showing tumour in left breast

History of scintimammography

In 1976, the first report of a radiotracer being taken up by a carcinoma occurred when it was noted that thallium-201 (being used to image the heart of a 47 year old man) was also taken up in the lung. Subsequently, the patient was later found to have bronchial carcinoma and a brief report of the case as a "complication of heart scintigraphy" appeared in the *British Journal of Radiology*.[2]

However, thallium's lack of sensitivity and specificity hindered further breast cancer imaging. Various radiopharmaceuticals were investigated including gallium-67 citrate, ^{99m}Tc-pertechnetate, the ^{99m}Tc-labelled phosphonates and ^{99m}Tc diethylene triamine penta-acetic acid (DTPA)[1] but they did not increase the specificity or sensitivity above the levels obtained with mammography.

However, in 1989, Muller and co-workers used a cardiac agent ^{99m}Tc sestamibi to image tumours in the lung. Localised areas of increased ^{99m}Tc sestamibi uptake were observed in 10 patients with untreated malignant tumours and research began into using ^{99m}Tc sestamibi specifically for imaging breast cancer. Previously, ^{99m}Tc sestamibi had been widely used in cardiovascular imaging for more than a decade. Research into the sensitivity, specificity and safety of ^{99m}Tc sestamibi in cardiovascular disease has been extensive.

As ^{99m}Tc sestamibi was developed originally to image the heart, cardiac uptake is high. Initially, this obscured any cancers highlighted against the chest area. The problem was solved by Khalkhali and co-workers[3] who imaged their patients in a prone position with the camera adjacent to the breast to separate the dependent breast from the chest wall. Other studies were then undertaken using ^{99m}Tc sestamibi to increase the technique's sensitivity and specificity. [4] (Table 1)

● [99m]Tc sestamibi was originally used as a cardiac imaging agent
● [99m]Tc sestamibi is now the radiopharmaceutical of choice in breast cancer imaging

Table 1 Scintimammography using ^{99m}Tc sestamibi

Principles of effective ^{99m}Tc sestamibi scintimammography

^{99m}Tc sestamibi scintimammography is a painless, non-invasive, nuclear medicine technique for the imaging of breast tissue. The radiopharmaceutical, sestamibi (Figure 2) is injected intravenously. As cancer cells tend to be more metabolically active than the healthy cells surrounding them, they take up more of the radiopharmaceutical. Indeed, uptake of sestamibi in cancer cells is nine times greater than in normal cells.[5] The radiopharmaceutical emits invisible gamma rays and a gamma camera is used to acquire lateral and anterior images of the breast for evaluation. Cancer is seen as focal areas of uptake on the scintimammogram.

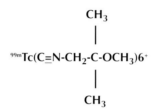

$$CH_3$$
$$|$$
$$^{99m}Tc(C{\equiv}N\text{-}CH_2\text{-}C\text{-}OCH_3)6^+$$
$$|$$
$$CH_3$$

Figure 2 ^{99m}Tc sestamibi molecule

Mechanism of uptake

The mechanism of uptake of ^{99m}Tc sestamibi is only partially understood. (Table 2)

- ^{99m}Tc sestamibi is taken up by cancer cells by an active transport mechanism and stored in the mitochondria and cytoplasm
- There appears to be a dynamic component of efflux of ^{99m}Tc sestamibi from cancer cells
- The rate of efflux is related to the expression of the MDR-1 gene and the cellular content of Pgp

Table 2   Uptake and efflux of ^{99m}Tc sestamibi

The influx of sestamibi into the cell is by an "active transport mechanism" and it appears to be stored in the mitochondria and the cytoplasm of the cancer cells.[6] As more mitochondria occur in metabolically active cancer cells than in surrounding normal tissue, ^{99m}Tc sestamibi accumulates in cancer cells. (Figure 3) As a result of this active transport mechanism, the images obtained are related to the metabolic activity of the cancer and not necessarily carcinoma size.

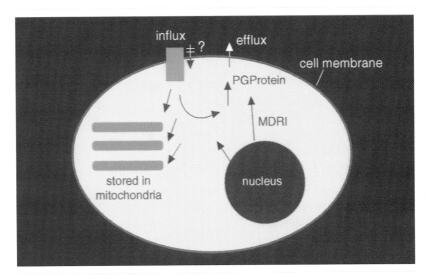

Figure 3   Uptake of sestamibi into tumour cells

Mechanisms of efflux

A number of factors appear to regulate efflux of ^{99m}Tc sestamibi from tumour cells. A dynamic component of efflux actively removes ^{99m}Tc sestamibi from the mitochondria and cytoplasm.[6,7] At least one mechanism appears to be linked to the gene known as the multi-drug resistance gene-1 (MDR-1). This has been studied because of its involvement in the development of resistance by various tumours to chemotherapeutic drugs.[8] [99m]Tc sestamibi is a substrate of P-glycoprotein (Pgp) which is encoded by MDR-1 and which appears to actively transport it out of tumour cells.[9] The rate of efflux is related to the expression of the MDR-1 gene and the cellular content of Pgp.[6,9] This expulsion of ^{99m}Tc sestamibi from cancer cells may prove useful in determining the response of a tumour to chemotherapy.

[99m]Tc sestamibi is excreted from the body via the hepatobiliary system and the kidneys. Eating after the injection and imaging procedure can accelerate the emptying of radiotracer from the gall-bladder.

Clinical results of ^{99m}Tc sestamibi scintimammography

Scintimammography with ^{99m}Tc sestamibi has been evaluated in single centre and multi-centre trials to assess its accuracy, sensitivity and specificity in both palpable and non-palpable lesions.

For example, a single centre study compared the accuracy of ^{99m}Tc sestamibi scintimammography with MRI and mammography.[10] It included 56 patients with suspect lesions detected by palpation or mammography. Of the lesions, 43 were palpable and 13 were non-palpable but were detected by mammography. Breast cancer was confirmed in 27 patients by histopathology with tumour sizes ranging from 6mm to 80mm in diameter. Scintimammography detected 23 breast cancers. There were four false-negative results. The sensitivity of all three techniques was similar although the specificity of scintimammography was much higher than either mammography or MRI. The sensitivity of scintimammography was also higher in palpable rather than non-palpable lesions. The diagnostic accuracy of the three evaluation techniques is given in Table 3.

Khalkhali et al[4] also assessed the sensitivity and specificity of ^{99m}Tc sestamibi scintimammography in a study involving 147 women with 153 lesions which required either breast biopsy or fine needle aspiration cytology. Of these, 113 were palpable and 40 were non-palpable. Reports from the scintimammography returned 47 true-positive and 11 false-positive lesions with 91 true-negative and four false-negative. These results were all confirmed by histopathology. The sensitivity of scintimammography in this study was 92.2% with a specificity of

	Scintimammography (%)	Mammography (%)	MRI (%)
Sensitivity	85	89	93
Specificity	66	14	21
Positive predictive value	70	49	52
Negative predictive value	83	57	75

Table 3   Overall diagnostic accuracy of scintimammography, mammography and MRI.[10]

89.2%.   A high positive predictive value of 81% and high negative predictive value of 95.8% was also recorded.

A large study involving 673 patients was conducted involving 42 clinical centres.[11-15] Randomised scintigraphic images were read by two groups of three blinded readers. Uptake was scored as either normal (no uptake), equivocal, low, moderate or high. The results were compared to histopathological results obtained from excisional biopsy. (Table 4)

[99m]Tc sestamibi in lesions <1cm and >1cm

In this multi-centre study, the sensitivity and specificity of any degree of uptake of ^{99m}Tc sestamibi was size-dependent and was much higher when the lesion was >1cm. This reflects the resolution possible with modern gamma cameras which is about 1cm as smaller objects (<1cm) may not be seen. For lesions <1cm, scintimammography may be of less use than MRI. In lesions ≥1cm, there is no significant difference in the sensitivity of scintimammography and MRI but the specificity of scintimammography is better. Since the readers in the multi-centre trial were blinded to the results of clinical examination, it is thought that specificity may be improved if scintimammography is read in conjunction with other clinical results such as patient histories and mammography. [11-15]

	Blinded image interpretation (%) (median values)	
Sensitivity	Palpable lesions	76
	Non-palpable lesions	52
Specificity	Palpable lesions	85
	Non-palpable lesions	94
Positive predictive value	Palpable lesions	83
	Non-palpable lesions	79
Negative predictive value	Palpable lesions	85
	Non-palpable lesions	94

Data from two multi-centre trials involving 673 patients.[11-15]

Table 4   The clinical accuracy of sestamibi scintimammography

Further analysis showed that diagnostic accuracy was similar in women with dense and fatty breasts compared with women with normal breast densities, independent of the size of the tumour. As a result, the authors concluded that the specificity and sensitivity of scintimammography is independent of breast density.

Other radiopharmaceuticals used in scintimammography

^{99m}Tc-labelled methylene diphosphonate (^{99m}Tc-MDP)

^{99m}Tc-MDP is used in bone imaging. In breast cancer imaging, it accurately detects carcinomas with diameters >10mm.[6,16]   However, the accumulation of ^{99m}Tc-MDP in cancerous tissue compared with surrounding tissue is less than is obtained using ^{99m}Tc sestamibi. The reported specificity and sensitivity varies depending on the patients recruited for the study but are lower than those for ^{99m}Tc sestamibi in most studies. (Figure 4)   Nevertheless, ^{99m}Tc-MDP may be valuable if the patient is also referred for bone scintigraphy.[6]

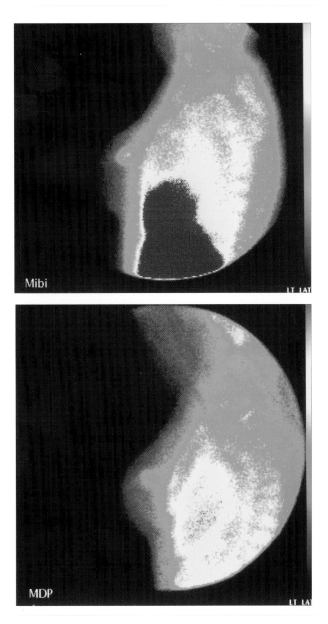

Figure 4   Images taken of the same patient showing comparative uptake of sestamibi and MDP

²⁰¹Tl-chloride

²⁰¹Tl-chloride (²⁰¹Tl) is possibly the simplest metabolic tumour marker in use because it is readily available and produces good tumour images using a planar gamma camera. However, its physical characteristics (long half-life and low energy radiation) mean that an initial dose of only 110 MBq may effectively produce a radiation dose to the patient as high as 25 mSV. Initial studies using the tracer were encouraging although it has been shown that uptake of ²⁰¹Tl is similar in both malignant and benign tumours.[6]

⁹⁹ᵐTc-tetrofosmin

⁹⁹ᵐTc-tetrofosmin is another agent produced for myocardial imaging that has been shown to image breast cancer in initial trials. However, the shortage of objective, controlled, multi-centre studies in this area make comparisons between agents difficult.

KEY POINTS

● Scintimammography can provide complementary images for use in the evaluation of breast cancers

● Various radiopharmaceuticals can be used in scintimammography but ⁹⁹ᵐTc sestamibi has emerged as the agent of choice due to its high sensitivity and specificity

● ⁹⁹ᵐTc sestamibi is taken up and expelled from tumour cells via an active transport mechanism. Efflux is dependent on a number of issues including the involvement of the MDR-1 gene and this may prove useful in determining a patient's response to chemotherapy

Chapter Four

The clinical role of scintimammography

The clinical role of scintimammography

Scintimammography as an aid to mammographic diagnosis

Scintimammography with ^{99m}Tc sestamibi can provide unique informa-tion for the diagnosis of breast cancer where it is recommended as a second line test following mammography. It is particularly useful where the mammogram is difficult to assess (e.g. where the breasts are dense and the mammogram is equivocal) or where compression of the breast required for mammography causes pain.

Difficult-to-evaluate mammograms

Dense breasts
The reading of mammograms of younger women with dense breasts is difficult. (Figure 1) The problem is common, occurring in about 25% of women under the age of 50.[1] In addition, the use of hormone replace-

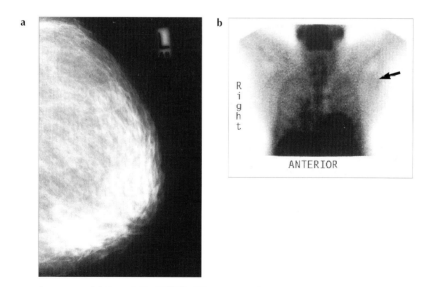

a   b

R
i
g
h
t

ANTERIOR

Figure 1   Image of (a) difficult mammogram - dense breast and
(b) a scintimammogram showing cancer as arrowed

ment therapy has added to the problem. Meanwhile, some herbal teas and Ginseng contain proto-oestrogens which may cause similar increases in the density of the breasts. These phenomena are particularly relevant in patients of East Asian origin who often use such agents. The addition of scintimammography with ^{99m}Tc sestamibi often overcomes the problem of the equivocal results of a mammogram in such women.

Breast implants

Silicone/saline breast implants are radio-opaque appearing as solid white masses on mammography. As a result, large portions of breast tissue are obscured even when special compression techniques are used. Scintimammography visualises any lesion within the breast tissue in these cases. (Figure 2)

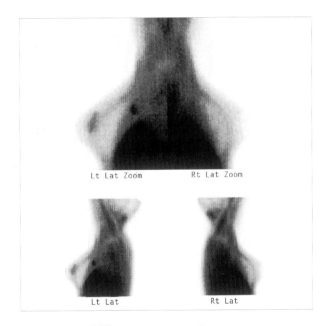

Figure 2   Scintimammography showing cancer in left breast of patient with subpectoral cosmetic implant

Lumpy breasts

Scintimammography is also valuable in patients with lumpy breasts who may undergo a series of mammograms. Such patients often undergo subsequent biopsy to investigate suspicious lesions which may itself lead to scarring making further interpretation of mammography difficult. If a biopsy is equivocal or negative, the addition of a negative ^{99m}Tc sestamibi study provides reassurance about the diagnosis.

Previous scarring or therapy

Mammograms are also difficult to interpret in patients who have undergone chemotherapy, radiation therapy or surgery for previous breast cancer. Post-surgical distortion may be caused by fibrosis, scarring, fat necrosis or focal lymph collection. Scintimammography has an important role to play in diagnosing recurrence in these patients where mammography is often unsatisfactory. The number of recurring breast lesions in patients who have undergone wide surgical excision is about 5%[2] and early identification of recurrence is clinically important for successful surgery.

Family history and genetic predisposition

A strong family history or genetic predisposition to breast cancer is an important risk factor, especially in first-degree relatives. It is important that these women are aware of this risk and check their breasts regularly. Screening mammography is usually undertaken after the age of 50 but in this group of patients it may be done at an earlier age than the screening population. This is usually when the women are in their 30s and 40s. At this age, their breasts tend to be more dense and mammography is often unsuitable. ^{99m}Tc scintimammography can be of use in identifying cancers which may be difficult to detect by mammography in these women.

Scintimammography as a qualitative test

Mammography is a qualitative test for breast cancer which depends on identifying subtle abnormal patterns within the breast architecture. In contrast, scintimammography is semi-quantitative showing either uptake or no uptake of the radiopharmaceutical. It is the presence of a focal uptake which indicates a cancer. In some patients with marked non-homogeneous breast tissue, the uptake of ^{99m}Tc sestamibi in the breast may itself be patchy. However, if no cancer is present, then focal uptake should also be absent. When this data is added to that collected from clinical examination, mammography and/or ultrasonography, ^{99m}Tc sestamibi scintimammography can help in making the diagnosis of cancer.

Scintimammography is not a substitute for mammography or biopsy. It should be used as a complementary test where other tests have produced equivocal results about the diagnosis or the nature of a suspicious lesion. Algorithms for incorporating scintimammography with ^{99m}Tc sestamibi into clinical protocols are discussed in a later chapter.

Scintimammography in the assessment of breast cancer

Scintimammography with ^{99m}Tc sestamibi is valuable in assessing the extent of breast cancer, particularly where there is multi-focal or bilateral disease which may not be fully diagnosed by mammography. It can also be used to clarify the extent of the disease in the breast where clinical and mammographic findings do not correspond.

Multi-centric and multi-focal disease
Mammography often fails to detect multi-centric or multi-focal breast cancer. It may underestimate the extent of the disease and only the main tumour mass may be recognised, especially where there is no significant calcification. This can lead to initial treatment failure. In such a case, scintimammography can show the full extent of the disease (Figure 3) allowing correct treatment to be planned. Scintimammography provides additional information about the location and dissemination of the cancer.

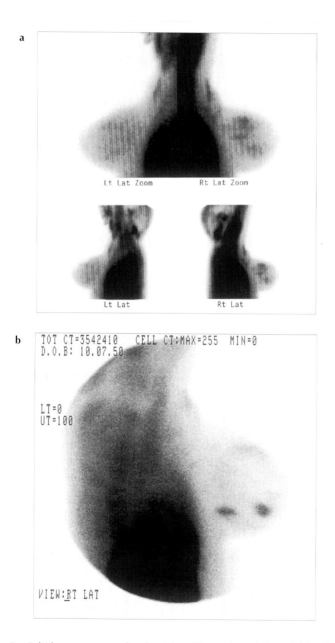

a

Lt Lat Zoom   Rt Lat Zoom

Lt Lat   Rt Lat

b

TOT CT=3542410   CELL CT:MAX=255 MIN=0
D.O.B: 10.07.50

LT=0
UT=100

VIEW:RT LAT

Figure 3   Scintimammograms showing (a) multi-centric and (b) multi-focal cancers

^{99m}Tc sestamibi scintimammography may be particularly useful as a diagnostic tool.

- Equivocal or non-diagnostic mammogram

- Dense or lumpy breasts

- Breast with distorting scars from previous surgery

- Recurrent breast cancer where there has been breast conserving surgery or there is scar tissue

- Breast implants

- Where mammography is difficult to undertake or where breast compression is too painful for the patient

- Strong family history of breast cancer where patients carry a genetic marker for the disease and where there is a need for further diagnostic information

- Hormone replacement therapy (HRT)

- Suspected multi-centric or multi-focal disease

- Palpable mass which is negative or equivocal at biopsy

- Dense mass without calcification

- Suspected multi-focal, multi-centric or bilateral disease

- Cases of suspected axillary lymph node involvement (ipsilateral and contralateral)

- Where the clinical extent of cancer is at variance with the mammographic findings

- Determining sites for biopsy (including ultrasound guided biopsy)

Axillary node involvement

When staging breast cancer, it is important to assess the degree of lymph node involvement which affects the prognosis and subsequent management. ^{99m}Tc sestamibi scintimammography can be used to view the axillary nodes and assess the spread of the disease. (Figure 4) The sensitivity for this technique ranges from 75-84.2% with specificity ranging from 90.9%-92.3%.[3-5] However, scintimammography should not be used alone to determine the presence or absence of lymph node involvement. If lymph node uptake is seen, it should be pursued by relevant biopsy. Additionally with scintimammography, but not sentinel node localisation, lymph node disease outside the main axillary lymph node groups can be identified. Thus, scintimammography can identify cancer in the internal mammary chain and infra- and supra-clavicular lymph nodes.

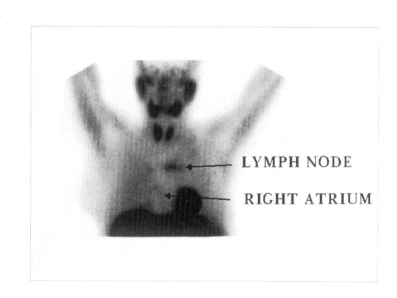

Figure 4 *Scintimammogram showing spread of disease into internal mammary lymph nodes*

Guiding biopsies

It is important when performing a biopsy that the correct location of the lesion is known and the aspiration material is extracted from the suspect area. ^{99m}Tc sestamibi using SPECT imaging can accurately locate cancer within the breast, even if it is situated close to the chest wall. Scintimammography can help the surgeon by guiding the biopsy to the abnormality within the breast to ensure that samples for cytology and histology are taken from the correct site.

The benefits of scintimammography

Benefits of scintimammography for the physician

● Complementary information for diagnosis and management
● Increased certainty of diagnosis where the mammogram is equivocal
● Alternative procedure when other imaging techniques are either inadequate, inappropriate or unavailable
● Planning of surgical intervention by providing detailed localisation of the lesion and its extent
● Identification of previously unsuspected secondary involvement either in the same breast, opposite breast or draining areas to identify multi-focal or multi-centric cancers previously missed on a mammogram
● Easy and simple technique using existing cameras

Benefits of scintimammography for the patient

● Non-invasive, non-compression imaging
● Increased certainty of diagnosis
● Convenient and painless

Quick and simple technique

Scintimammography offers existing modern nuclear medicine departments opportunities to improve the diagnosis of breast cancer without the need for expensive new equipment or time-consuming techniques. The procedure is quick and simple and the results are available to the clinician immediately for assessment. As a result, periods of anxiety can be reduced. Scintimammography is a painless procedure which is well tolerated by most patients. Unlike mammography, scintimammography does not require the compression of the breast which many women find uncomfortable.

Complementary information

Women undergoing tests for breast cancer often suffer anxiety and stress when they are recalled due to an equivocal mammogram. The availability of scintimammography offers a quick and painless imaging technique which can help to alleviate their fears by providing the additional information for a more certain diagnosis. It also particularly provides an alternative technique where other imaging techniques are unsatisfactory.

Accurate surgical planning

Scintimammography provides surgeons and oncologists with useful information about the extent and location of breast cancer. As surgery needs to excise sufficient breast tissue to eliminate the disease or to allow for further non-surgical treatment, information obtained by scintimammography can highlight the full extent of cancer within the breast. Thus, treatments, including surgery, can be planned more accurately from the start.

Identification of full extent of disease

Scintimammography can give information about the true nature of multi-centric, multi-focal and bilateral cancer which may not be available from other imaging techniques. These data can be used to tailor treatment strategies for the particular patient.

Case studies using scintimammography

Clinical applications showing examples of
patients' images and brief case histories

Case 1

**Patient history
and examination:** 45 year old pre-menopausal
patient with three week history
of right breast lump. Clinical
carcinoma (40 x 50mm)
LOQ right breast

Mammography: Right breast carcinoma

Clinical problem: Patient suitable for primary
cytotoxic chemotherapy.
Does the carcinoma show on
scintimammography and can
this be used to assess response?

Scintimammography: Showed additional focus of carcinoma
not identified on initial mammography

Histopathology: Grade II invasive ductal carcinoma and
in situ ductal carcinoma

**Impact of
scintimammography on
diagnosis and management:** In view of multi-centric carcinoma,
patient underwent total mastectomy
following clinical response. Mastectomy
showed residual *in situ* disease but no
invasive component

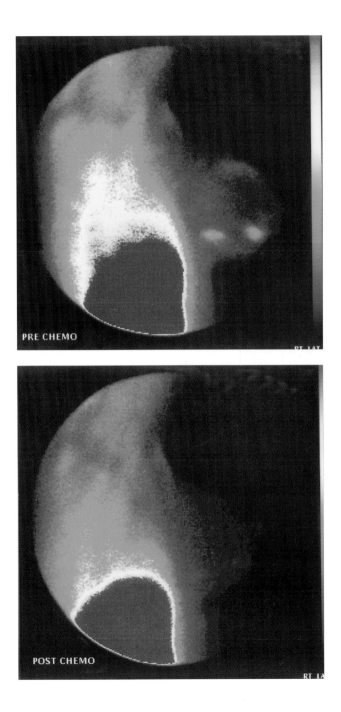

Case 2

Patient history and examination:
46 year old post-menopausal woman presented with a painful lump in the left breast. Her sister had died of breast cancer at the age of 32. The left breast was larger with slight nipple inversion. Three nodules were noted in three different quadrants. Clinical fibrocystic change was suspected

Mammography:
Dense breast tissue was noted. Extensive microcalcification was noted in the LIQ

Clinical problem:
The family history and nipple inversion as well as microcalcification on mammography were suspicious features. FNA of the three lumps and a blind biopsy of the area of microcalcification were carried out

Scintimammography:
Showed four quadrant uptake in the breast and left axillary nodes

Histopathology:
Cytology showed high grade carcinoma in all four quadrants. Mastectomy specimen showed Grade III invasive ductal and *in situ* carcinoma. Eighteen axillary nodes involved

Impact of scintimammography on diagnosis and management:
Showed true extent of carcinoma and metastatic disease. Patient therefore underwent total mastectomy and axillary clearance followed by high dose cytotoxic adjuvant chemotherapy

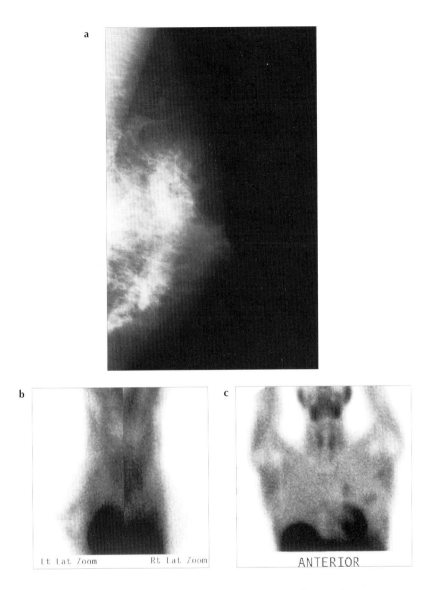

(a) Left mammogram shows increased irregular densities with extensive microcalcification
(b and c) Lateral and anterior scintimammographic views show multi-centric focal uptake and uptake in left axillary nodes

Case 3

History and examination:	56 year old patient presented with a clinical carcinoma (T3NOMO) of the left breast. Cytology confirmed carcinoma
Medication:	Had been taking hormone replacement therapy for two and a half years but stopped on finding lump
Mammography:	Localised tissue density in the medial segment of the left breast. The mammogram was reported as showing no specific features
Clinical problem:	Since mammography had not shown a definite lesion, scintimammography was ordered to assess the extent of the tumour and any other impalpable lesions which would have changed management
Scintimammography:	Focal uptake left breast. No other uptake in rest of breast or opposite breast. Slight focal uptake in left axillary nodes
Histology:	Grade II invasive ductal carcinoma + Grade III DCIS
Impact of scintimammography on assessment and management:	Provided local extent of carcinoma to be treated by primary cytotoxic chemotherapy. Scintimammography used to assess extent of residual tumour bulk following chemotherapy
Follow-up:	Good clinical response to cytotoxic chemotherapy. Scintimammography showed small area of residual activity at site of original cancer. Both area and activity of sestamibi markedly reduced

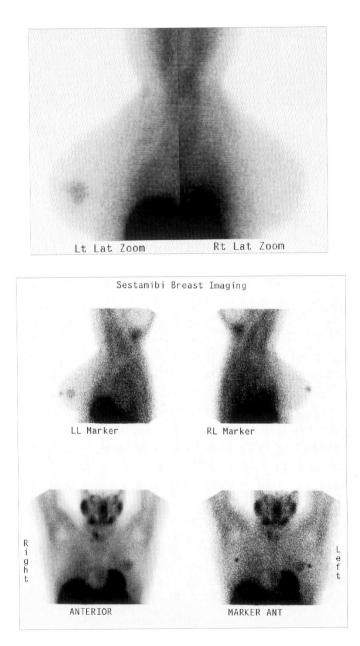

Focal uptake left breast. No other uptake in rest of breast or opposite breast. Slight focal uptake in left axillary nodes

Case 4

History and examination: 47 year old patient presented with recent onset of right inflammatory breast cancer. No response to primary chemotherapy using a doxorubicin regimen. Some response - tumour shrinkage following three doses of taxoid

Past history: Left mastectomy

Clinical problem: Oedema and persisting erythema of the breast made accurate evaluation of response difficult. Mammogram too dense to separate carcinoma residue from oedematous breast

Scintimammography: Clearly defined uptake indicating major tumour residue and involved axillary nodes

Histology: Pleomorphic high grade carcinoma with areas of necrosis, inflammation and vascular invasion

Impact of scintimammography on assessment and management: Residual carcinoma clearly seen. Depth of carcinoma shown on scintimammography confirmed by histology and inflammatory type indicated post-mastectomy radiotherapy to chest wall. Extensive uptake in axillary nodes despite two types of cytotoxic chemotherapy indicated surgical axillary clearance

Follow-up: Patient is on adjuvant tamoxifen

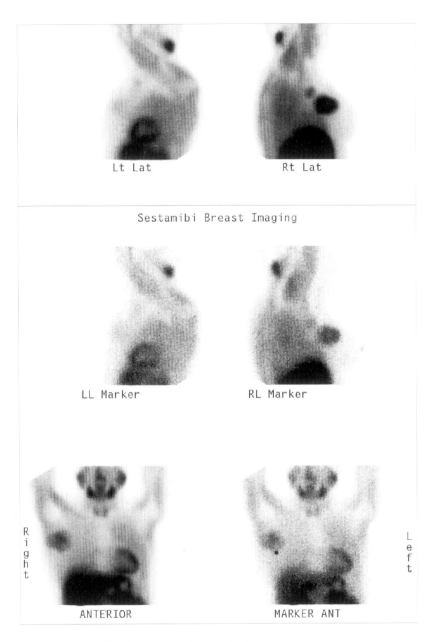

Lt Lat | Rt Lat

Sestamibi Breast Imaging

LL Marker | RL Marker

Right | Left

ANTERIOR | MARKER ANT

Scintimammography after course of cytotoxic chemotherapy

Case 5

Patient history and examination: 34 year old patient presented with a rapidly increasing right breast lump over four months. Clinical inflammatory carcinoma of breast with axillary involvement

Mammography: Both breasts are diffusely dense. On the right side a dense 8cm mass noted in centre of breast. Neoplasm suspected

Clinical problem: Clinical carcinoma but full extent unclear from mammography. Clinical extent may be misleading due to oedema of the breast

Scintimammography: Extensive focal uptake in right breast and axillary nodes. No uptake in left breast

Histopathology: Grade III invasive ductal carcinoma and comedo ductal carcinoma *in situ*. Oestrogen receptor poor

Impact of scintimammography on management: Initial and subsequent scintimammography provided better extent of carcinoma than mammography. Follow-up sestamibi scan showed residual carcinoma in keeping with partial clinical response to primary cytotoxic chemotherapy. Core biopsy showed residual carcinoma. Patient underwent total mastectomy and axillary clearance followed by adjuvant cytotoxic chemotherapy

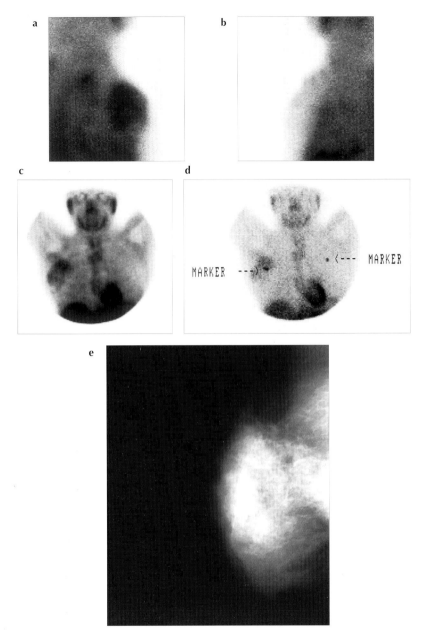

(a-d) Scintimammogram showing extensive uptake in right breast and axillary nodes
(e) Mammogram shows large dense suspicious mass

Case 6

History and examination:

In 1988 this 60 year old patient underwent a right segmental mastectomy and axillary clearance. She subsequently developed bone metastases and was treated with a series of hormonal agents. She was on aminoglutethimide with good initial control until January 1997 when the left breast became swollen, firmer but without a discrete mass. No clinical recurrence was noted in the right breast. There were significant nodes in both axillae and thickening in the left supraclavicular fossa but no nodes

Mammography:

Suspicious density and microcalcification in the left breast suggestive of a carcinoma

Scintimammography:

Uptake in both breasts and axillae

Liver ultrasound scan:

Hepatic metastases

Bone scan:

Progression of bone metastases

Follow-up:

Patient switched to cytotoxic chemotherapy

Impact of scintimammography on assessment and management:

The carcinoma in the left breast was impalpable and scintimammography indicated the extent. Clinical and mammographic examination failed to show recurrence in the right breast although this was suspected. Scintimammography provided a good baseline of the cancers in both breasts and axillae prior to instituting new therapy for locally advanced carcinoma

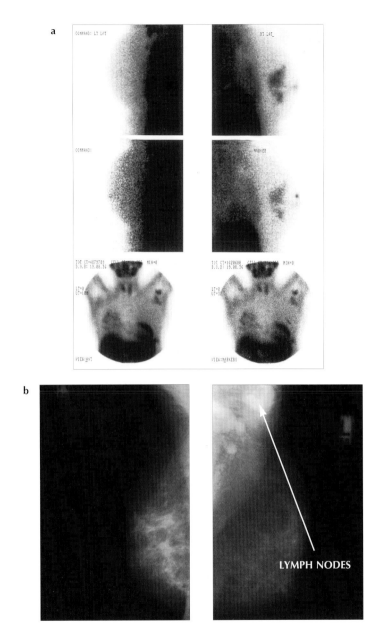

(a) *Scintimammography shows uptake in both breasts and axillae*
(b) *Right mammogram shows recurrent cancer. Left mammogram shows suspicious density and microcalcification and enlarged axillary lymph nodes*

Case 7

History and examination:	67 year old woman presented with a 40mm lump in right breast with skin changes. A 30mm mass of nodes felt in ipsilateral axilla. [T4N1M0]
Mammography:	Extensive infiltration of right breast by tumour
Cytology:	Carcinoma
Scintimammography:	Uptake in LOQ of right breast as well as focal uptake in right axilla. Depth of carcinoma well seen on lateral view
Surgery:	Total mastectomy and axillary clearance
Histology:	Grade II invasive ductal carcinoma extending to 1mm of pectoral fascia and involving skin anteriorly. Ten of 16 nodes showed metastatic carcinoma which was strongly oestrogen and progesterone positive
Adjuvant therapy:	Patient commenced on tamoxifen and referred for chest wall radiotherapy
Impact of scintimammography on assessment and management:	Primary carcinoma and axillary metastases clearly seen. Depth of carcinoma in relation to pectoral fascia seen on scintiscan. Since clinical picture and mammography indicated carcinoma and extent, scintimammography did not provide additional information to change management

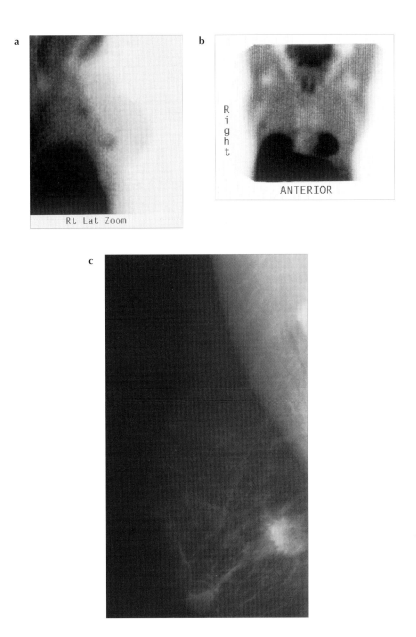

(a and b) Scintimammogram shows uptake in LOQ of right breast as well as focal uptake in right axilla. Depth of carcinoma well seen on lateral view
(c) Mammogram shows extensive infiltration of right breast by cancer

Case 8

History and examination:	Asymptomatic 55 year old patient had a UK Breast Screening Programme mammogram which showed extensive microcalcification in the left breast. There was no palpable lesion but "blind" fine needle aspiration biopsy of the upper central portion of the breast showed malignant cells
Family history:	No family history of breast cancer but her mother died from a primary glioma of the brain at the age of 48
Medication:	Patient had been on hormone replacement therapy for six years
Clinical problem:	Investigations did not clarify whether patient had invasive or *in situ* carcinoma. Extent of carcinoma not clearly defined
Scintimammography:	Multi-centric uptake in left breast
Histology:	Two primary invasive ductal carcinomas - one a Grade I (10mm) and the other Grade II (9x7mm diameter). Foci of cribriform and solid ductal carcinoma *in situ* were seen in and around the tumours. Three of fifteen nodes were involved. Immunochemistry showed strong diffuse staining for oestrogen and progesterone receptors
Impact of scintimammography on assessment and management:	In view of multi-centric uptake, extensive microcalcification and cytology, patient advised to have mastectomy and axillary clearance
Follow-up:	Patient has stopped hormone replacement therapy and is on adjuvant tamoxifen

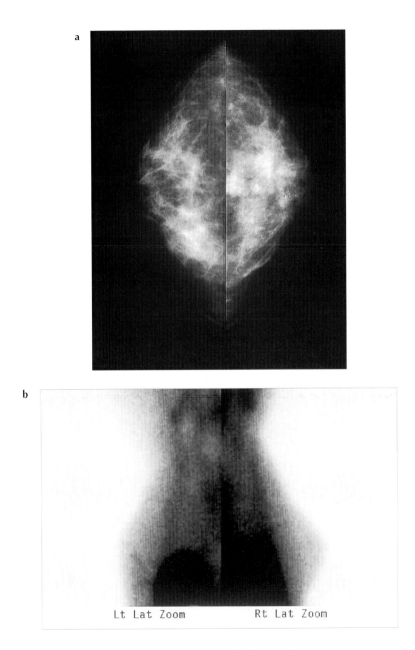

(a) *Mammogram shows extensive microcalcification in left breast*
(b) *Scintimammography shows multi-centric uptake in left breast*

Case 9

History and examination: A 60 year old patient presented with a clinical recurrent carcinoma of the left breast following wide local excision and radiotherapy. She was on adjuvant tamoxifen

Past history: Previous treatment for Hodgkin's lymphoma and endometrial carcinoma in forties

Clinical problem: Patient refused mastectomy although no other site of carcinoma was detected

Management: FNA cytology confirmed cancer. Tamoxifen stopped and megestrol acetate started with good response. After 12 months the patient appeared to have lost response - greater induration and oedema of left breast

Scintimammography: Uptake in left breast with improvement on megestrol acetate. Repeat scan at 12 months showed increased localised uptake in left breast

Histology: Core biopsy did not show carcinoma

Management: Patient preferred to change hormone manipulation rather than undergo mastectomy. Megestrol acetate stopped and anastrozole started

MRI scan with gadolinium enhancement: Tumour recurrence extending to pectoral fascia

Management: Patient to review option of mastectomy

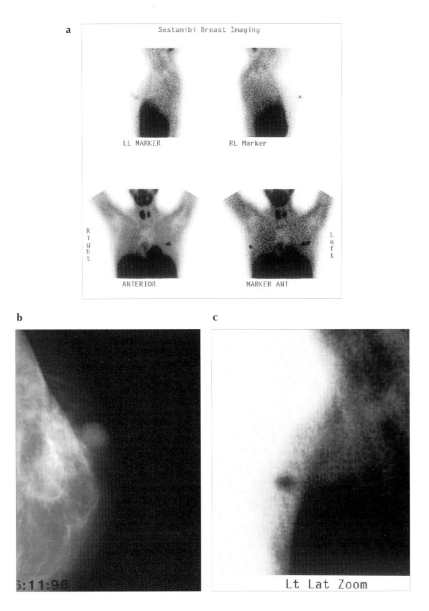

(a) Uptake in left breast
(b) Mammogram shows extensive scarring but no clear evidence of recurrence
(c) Focal uptake in left breast on scintimammogram

Case 10 - Local recurrence after mastectomy

History and examination: 70 year old obese patient who had undergone a right total mastectomy. Tumour marker CA 153 raised. Clinical examination - no recurrent disease. Biochemical tests, chest X-ray and abdominal scans showed no metastases. Fullness upper mastectomy flap. FNA x 2 - ve

Mammography: No abnormality in left breast

Clinical problem: Markedly raised CA 153 (600) without evidence of recurrence

Scintimammography: Uptake in upper mastectomy flap. No uptake in left breast

Impact of scintimammography on management and outcome: Patient started on cytotoxic and then hormonal chemotherapy with excellent response - clinical improvement and fall in CA 153 to 68 within five months

Learning point: Sestamibi scintiscanning may have a special role in the identification and targeting of site of subcutaneous local recurrence in obese patients

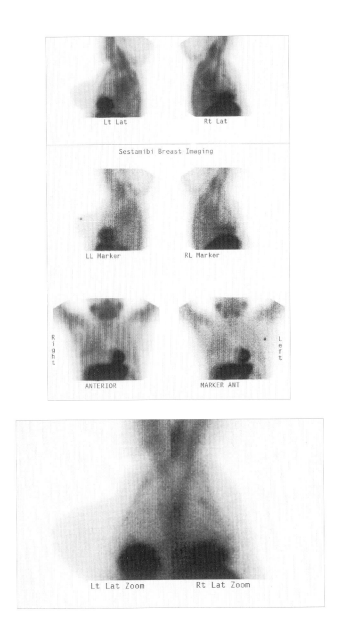

Uptake in fat of right upper mastectomy flap

Case 11

History and examination:

59 year old patient with previous local surgery and radiotherapy for carcinoma of the breast presented with thyroid swelling - ? thyroid carcinoma to ENT surgeon who found metastatic breast carcinoma. Examination showed fibrotic left upper chest wall ? radiation change or recurrent cancer

Clinical problem:

Patient with known neck and bone metastases but breast and chest wall disease unclear

Scintimammography:

No breast uptake but uptake in left chest wall in radiotherapy field. During therapy with tamoxifen noted distortion of right breast. Scintimammography showed no uptake in breasts confirming negative findings on mammography. Scan still showed some uptake in left upper chest wall

Impact of scintiscanning on assessment and management:

Scintimammography showed site and extent of chest wall recurrence suspected clinically. We were able to reassure patient about the right breast

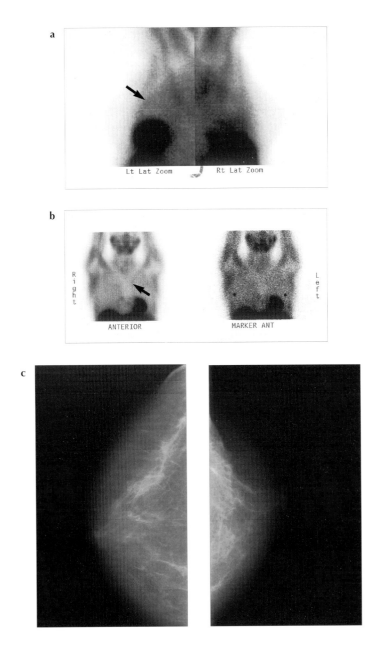

(a and b) Scintimammography
(c) Mammography showed no evidence of recurrence

Case 12

History and examination:	Gynaecologist had noticed slightly nodular area in lower left breast in 42 year old patient on routine check and referred patient to a breast surgeon. No discrete mass on examination
Ultrasound breast scan:	No discrete lesion
Mammogram:	Dense breasts. No discrete lesion reported
MRI:	Suspicious lesion on lower left breast
Scintimammography:	Focal uptake in lower left breast
Core biopsy histology:	Ductal carcinoma *in situ* (DCIS)
Excision biopsy of area of sestamibi uptake:	DCIS to margin of biopsy
Consultation:	Patient advised to undergo total mastectomy and immediate reconstruction. Patient opted for mastectomy and consideration of reconstruction at a later date
Histology of mastectomy:	Focus of residual DCIS. No invasive carcinoma
Follow-up:	No adjuvant treatment required. Annual follow-up to assess right breast

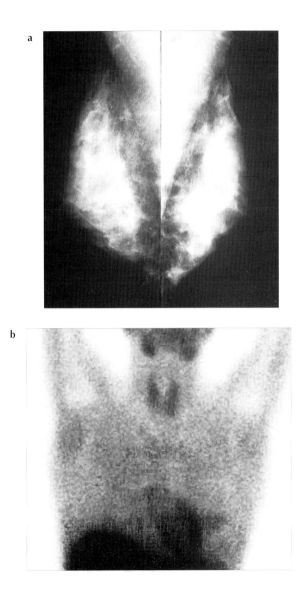

(a) Mammogram showing dense breasts
(b) Scintimammogram shows uptake in lower left breast

When is scintimammography inappropriate?

[99m]Tc sestamibi scintimammography is suitable for most patients. However, it is inappropriate for technical or safety reasons in a small number of patients. These include women with diseases of the spine; very obese patients who may be unable to lie prone for the required acquisition times; those suffering from claustrophobia who may be unable to tolerate the proximity of the camera; and, pregnant patients.

KEY POINTS

- Scintimammography is a useful second line imaging procedure for the diagnosis and evaluation of the location and extent of breast cancer
- [99m]Tc sestamibi scintimammography is especially useful in patients with mammographically dense breasts, post-surgical or post-radiation breast changes and women on hormone replacement therapy or with breast implants
- [99m]Tc sestamibi scintimammography is also valuable in the assessment of breast cancer including involvement of axillary nodes
- Both patients and physicians can benefit from using ^{99m}Tc sestamibi scintimammography in diagnostic and assessment protocols
- Scintimammography is suitable for most women

Chapter Five

Performing high quality
scintimammography with ^{99m}Tc sestamibi

Performing high quality scintimammography with ^{99m}Tc sestamibi

Equipment needed

Scintimammography is a simple procedure which can be undertaken in most community hospitals equipped with a modern nuclear medicine department. Existing gamma cameras (double or single headed) can be used to acquire images. The gamma camera need not be new but it should be well maintained with good intrinsic resolution and good uniformity and a high resolution collimator is essential. Double headed cameras require less repositioning of the patient.

An imaging couch is required with specially designed breast "cut-outs" to allow the breasts to be fully dependent. (Figure 1)

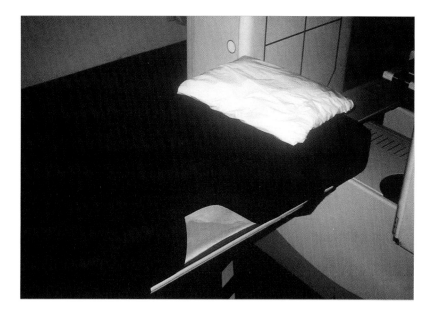

Figure 1   *Gamma camera and imaging couch showing breast "cut-outs"*

Good quality control is essential in the preparation of the radiophar-maceutical, the injection and the imaging procedure to ensure acquisition of optimal images.

Since there is no compression of the breast, no special equipment is needed apart from the imaging couch. The procedure is convenient for both the department and the patients as both breasts can be imaged at the same time.

Preparing the radiopharmaceutical and injection into the patient

Sestamibi can be prepared simply and quickly in any radiopharmacy from pyrogen-free vials and ^{99m}Tc pertechnetate. It may take a radiopharmacist or nuclear imaging technician up to 40 minutes to prepare and should be prepared in accordance with the manufacturer's instructions. Hospital quality control protocols for the administration of pharmaceuticals to patients should be followed. Records should be kept of the radioactivity dispensed to the patient. Activity (allowing for decay) in a single vial is sufficient to perform four 750 MBq ^{99m}Tc sestamibi studies over a four hour period.

A dose of 740 MBq of ^{99m}Tc sestamibi (range 700-800 MBq) is injected into the patient followed by a 10-20mls saline flush into an available vein in the foot or arm contralateral to the breast being imaged. (Figure 2) Injections into the feet are preferred to reduce any leakage of radiopharmaceutical into surrounding tissues which may adversely affect the image. If the injection is given in the arm, it is important to get a "clean" injection to avoid artifactual axillary node uptake from extravasated ^{99m}Tc sestamibi via lymphatic drainage. As scintimammography images axillary nodes as well as the breast, it is important to be able to distinguish uptake associated with a lesion from uptake due to a tissued injection.

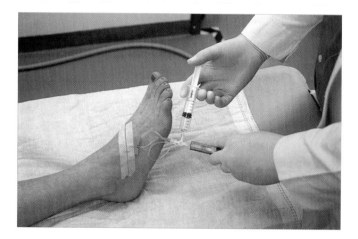

Figure 2   Foot injection

The patient is imaged within 5-10 minutes of the injection. Early studies reported that the radiopharmaceutical may be significantly washed out within an hour reducing the imaging potential.[1] Patients may experience a slight metallic taste after the injection but this will pass.

Imaging protocol

Scintimammography is a painless procedure which does not require compression of the breasts. However, women with spinal problems may experience some discomfort lying prone for extended periods of time. In these cases, it may be useful to allow the patients time to relax between the acquisition of images. (Table 1)

- Prepare radiopharmaceutical
- Inject radiopharmaceutical into vein in foot or contralateral arm
- Patient is imaged within 5-10 minutes of the injection
- Prone and lateral views of each breast are acquired for 10 minutes per view
- Nipple marker views are acquired for three minutes per view

Table 1   Imaging protocol

Imaging is undertaken with the woman lying prone with her head resting on her arms on a scintimammography mattress to allow the greatest separation of the breast from the myocardium and liver.[2] The breast to be imaged should be fully dependent (Figure 3) while the opposite breast may be dependent behind a specially-designed lead shield or compressed on the couch. This ensures that no "shine through" occurs.

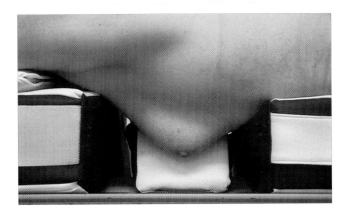

Figure 3   Patient in prone position

Imaging should be performed in a minimum 128 x 128 word matrix using an ultra high resolution or high resolution collimator. (Table 2)

- High resolution collimator
- 128 x 128 matrix
- 10-15% window centered on 140 keV
- Acquisition time: 10 minutes per view (three minutes per marker view)

Table 2   Acquisition parameters

Windows should be set at 10-15% around a 140 keV peak depending on the septal penetration of the collimators used (e.g. some foil collimators have significant shine through at 140 keV and a tighter 10% window is needed). The camera head should be as close as possible to the patient. (Figure 4)

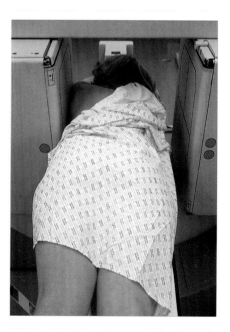

Figure 4   Camera head as close as possible to patient

As scintimammography does not provide any structural reference points, a cobalt 57 marker is used to identify the nipple on every image. (Figure 5)

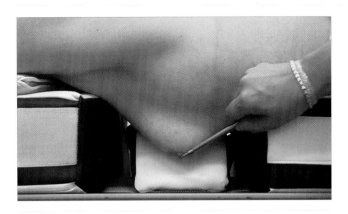

Figure 5   Image showing nipple marker views

Once prone lateral views of both breasts (if required) have been acquired, a supine anterior image is obtained. The patient lies supine with her arms raised above her head to provide a clear image of the axilla. (Figure 6) The anterior supine image is always acquired after the lateral images, as high lung uptake may initially obscure the breast images.

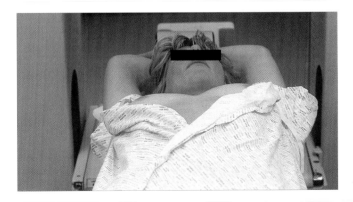

Figure 6   Patient in supine position

Views acquired

Six views are normally acquired (Figure 7):
- Prone right lateral breast for 10 minutes
- Prone right lateral breast with nipple marker for three minutes
- Prone left lateral breast for 10 minutes
- Prone left lateral breast with nipple marker for three minutes
- Supine anterior breasts for 10 minutes
- Supine anterior breasts with nipple markers for three minutes

Processing the data

Images are best read from computer screens for optimal intensity and contrast of the image while printed copies provide records and assessment. Initially, the three breast images are displayed and the maximum counts in normal breast tissue are noted. Truncating of maximum counts to the maximum in the breast or logarithmic scales should be used to ensure that activity in the breast is not swamped by activity from the chest wall. Different computer systems provide varying techniques and some experimentation should be undertaken to achieve optimal imaging. (Figure 8)

Single photon emission computed tomography (SPECT)

SPECT is used to gather images of "slices" of the chest through 360° around the patient. Each slice is taken for 30 seconds at selected intervals and images can be combined to provide a three-dimensional image of the chest providing valuable information about the location of any lesions for planning surgery. Indeed SPECT can give information about the precise location of the primary breast abnormality and also help to determine the presence of lymph node involvement of the axilla. (Figure 9)

SPECT images can be acquired using any tomographic gamma camera. Although experimental imaging has been performed using prone imaging in special SPECT cushions, high quality SPECT images can be achieved with the patient in the supine position with the woman's arms elevated above her head. SPECT may be most useful in finding lesions in the axillary tail and lymph node disease. Planar imaging is better at finding disease within the breast itself. Using a single headed gamma

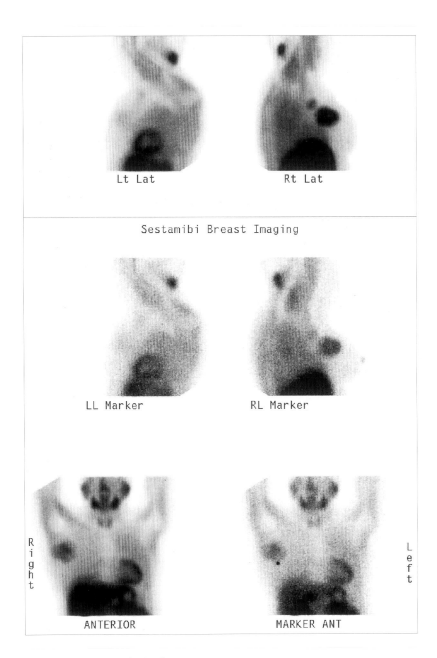

Figure 7   Six views obtained

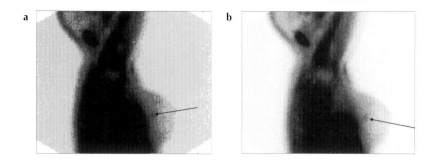

Figure 8   (a) non-truncated and (b) truncated images. The truncated image clearly shows the cancer is separated from the chest wall

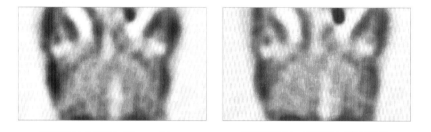

Figure 9   Coronal SPECT slices showing uptake in axillary lymph nodes bilaterally

camera, a 360° rotation is recommended with a minimum of 60 stops and 30 seconds per stop. This time can be adjusted in multi-headed gamma cameras.

SPECT images are viewed in cine mode and any corrections made for movements using motion correction software while sinogram can be useful in determining if motion has occurred. The data should then be reconstructed one pixel thick using a simple back-projection and smoothing filter. If available, iterative reconstruction should be used. From the main transaxial data set, orthogonal slices are then recon-structed in transaxial, sagittal and coronal slices. Images are best viewed on a computer where manipulation of the colour scale may be required to prevent high activity in the heart obscuring activity in tumours or metastatic lymph nodes.

Common pitfalls of imaging

Scintimammography is a simple technique to perform but, as with any nuclear medicine imaging, care must be taken to avoid simple pitfalls. (Table 3)

- Injection leakage
- Wrong positioning of patient or camera
- Incorrect acquisition times
- Incorrect assessment of normal uptake in the heart, thyroid and liver
- Couch scatter

Table 3   Common pitfalls of imaging

Leakage of injection

Leakage of the radiopharmaceutical into local tissue or the lymphatic system may affect the accuracy of the image obtained. (Figure 10) To avoid this, it is recommended that all injections are made via an available foot vein.

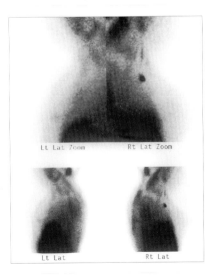

Figure 10 Image showing arm and false axillary uptake following leakage at site of arm injection

Wrong positioning of patient - breast not fully dependent

It is important to ensure that the breast to be imaged is not constricted by the imaging couch. The breast should be fully dependent and elongated by gravity. Incorrect positioning (Figure 11) will give sub-optimal images of the breast.

a

b

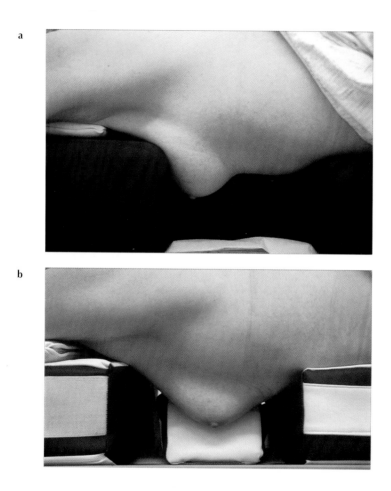

Figure 11 (a) incorrect and (b) correct patient positioning

Wrong positioning of camera

Cameras should be positioned as close as possible to the patient to ensure the best acquisition of the image. If patients feel claustrophobic, it may be preferable to use a single headed camera. (Figure 12)

a   b

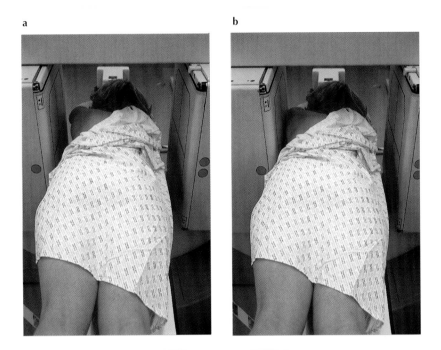

*Figure 12 The camera head in (a) is positioned too far away from the
patient compared to the correct position (b)*

Incorrect acquisition times

Acquisition times of 10 minutes per diagnostic view and three minutes per marker view are recommended. Insufficient acquisition time may result in a sub-optimal image.

Thyroid uptake which can mimic lymph node uptake

Sestamibi is known to be taken up by the thyroid gland which can clearly be seen on scintimammograms. Care must be taken when differentiating between lymph node uptake and thyroid uptake. (Figure 13)

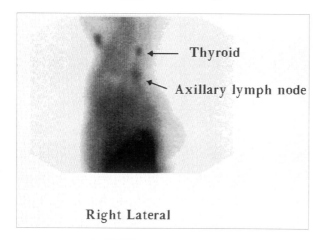

Figure 13 Example of thyroid uptake

Uptake in the heart

Since sestamibi was originally developed as a cardiac imaging agent, there is significant uptake in the heart and the liver. Readers should be aware of normal patterns of uptake when evaluating images. (Figure 14)

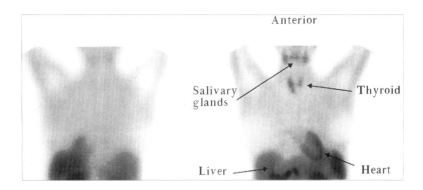

Figure 14 Example highlighting uptake in the heart and liver

Couch scatter/shine through

Couch scatter may affect the quality of the image and appear as diffuse or patchy uptake across the image. This may be particularly apparent if using metal and non carbon-fibre couches. There may also be diffuse or patchy uptake if the opposite breast is not properly shielded from the camera either by compression or the use of a lead shield. (Figure 15)

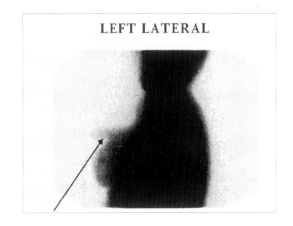

LEFT LATERAL

Figure 15 Shine through from poorly shielded right breast

Scar tissue

It is thought that a fresh haematoma may have some increased uptake of ^{99m}Tc sestamibi to a greater extent than normal tissue. Therefore, imaging is not recommended within seven days of an operation or biopsy. However, there is no evidence to suggest that scar tissue has an increased uptake of ^{99m}Tc sestamibi unless there is recurrence of cancer in the scar.

KEY POINTS

- Scintimammography is a simple technique which can be performed in most modern nuclear medicine departments without the need to buy specialist equipment
- Imaging takes approximately 40 minutes to one hour for six views to be obtained
- Care should be taken when administering the radiopharmaceutical and positioning the patient and camera to obtain the best images
- Images are best read from computer screens
- Interpretation of the results is simple but requires a knowledge of common pitfalls in order to avoid false positive results

Chapter Six

Incorporating scintimammography into the diagnosis and management of breast cancer

Incorporating scintimammography into the diagnosis and management of breast cancer

Introduction

The provision of healthcare services in most countries today is dependent on a number of factors including the need for the service, usefulness, cost and availability. It is, therefore, important that any new test or procedure is incorporated into management plans in a cost effective way where it can provide the most benefit to patients and doctors. Recommended management guidelines are now being used to optimise the treatment of many diseases, to decide on the best time to initiate tests and to guide therapy.

As the needs of cancer centres may differ greatly, it is important that ^{99m}Tc sestamibi scintimammography is placed in the correct clinical algorithm. This will vary from centre to centre depending on the availability and accuracy of other diagnostic tests. Examples of algorithms for patients with suspicious palpable breast lumps and those in whom mammography shows an impalpable lesion are seen in Figures 1 and 2. These algorithms also separate diagnostic procedures required after a positive or negative mammogram. In patients with equivocal mammograms scintimammography provides useful information.

For primary breast cancer

a) When mammography is positive

In those with a positive mammogram (Figure 1), the majority will not need scintimammography. However, when there is scarring in the breast or diffuse microcalcification, scintimammography would be helpful in deciding if biopsy is required. In those with other abnormalities of the mammograms, a core or localisation biopsy may be indicated. Scintimammography, however, may still be useful in those patients with larger tumours to determine if the tumour is multi-focal or multi-centric or in evaluating the extent of disease.

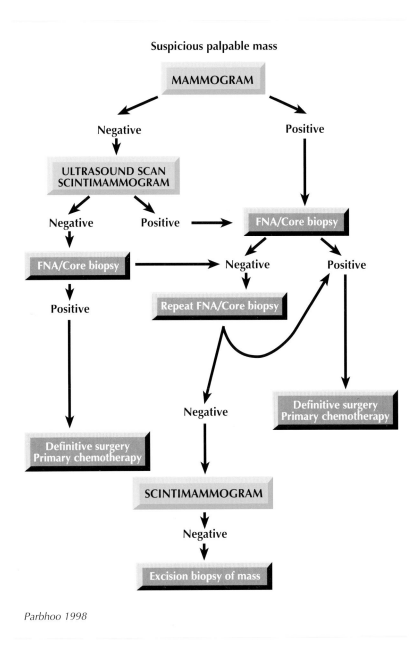

Suspicious palpable mass

Parbhoo 1998

Figure 1   Diagnostic algorithm for suspicious palpable breast lump

Scintimammography can also play a significant role in planning of surgery in women with known breast cancer. In patients where significant abnormalities are seen on an X-ray mammogram but the extent of cancer is unclear, scintimammography can determine the extent of cancer, whether it is attached to the chest wall and possible lymph node involvement. Additionally, multi-focal or multi-centric and primary, unsuspected cancers in the opposite breast may also be seen.

The data obtained can then be used to identify the best management. For example, it reduces the risk that the breast mass is removed without including the margins of the tumour which can result in the need for additional surgery. Scintimammography showing extensive cancer or multi-focal/centric disease allows definitive surgical treatment to be planned and discussed with the patient and her family prior to the procedure.

When screening mammography shows an impalpable lesion the diagnostic algorithm in Figure 2 is suggested. Small focal lesions will not be seen on scintimammography until the resolution of the gamma camera detectors improves. In large or diffuse lesions scintimammography may help in the decision process and in determining the extent of surgery.

b) When mammography is equivocal

Scintimammography is important in patients with suspected breast cancer and a non-diagnostic or equivocal mammogram. Selection of ultrasound or scintimammography is dependent on the local availability of equipment and skilled operators. Each technique provides complementary information but problems leading to difficulties with mammography may also render ultrasound less useful.

In patients with non-palpable masses which are <7-8mm, the sensitivity of scintimammography is insufficient to allow a negative test to be regarded as clinically definitive. Therefore, if cancer is still suspected in patients with negative scintimammographic studies, they should be considered for a more sensitive study such as MRI. However, it must be remembered that even using gadolinium wash-in and wash-out rates, the specificity of MRI of the breast may be as low as 20-40%.[1-3] These patients will require a stereotactic localisation biopsy.

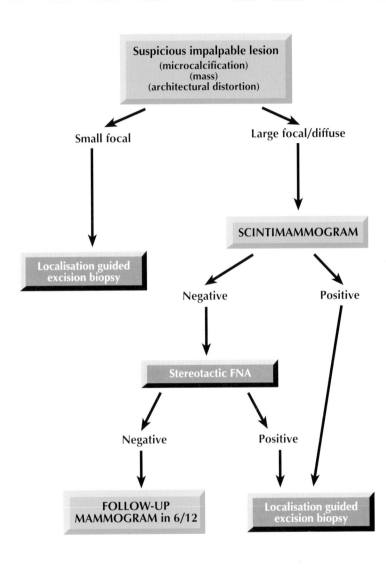

Suspicious impalpable lesion
(microcalcification)
(mass)
(architectural distortion)

Small focal

Large focal/diffuse

Localisation guided excision biopsy

SCINTIMAMMOGRAM

Negative

Positive

Stereotactic FNA

Negative

Positive

FOLLOW-UP MAMMOGRAM in 6/12

Localisation guided excision biopsy

Parbhoo 1998

Figure 2 *Diagnostic algorithm for impalpable lesion seen on X-ray mammogram*

c) When the mammogram is negative

In those patients with a negative mammogram (Figure 1) the next test is normally an ultrasound of the breast. Palpable cysts identified on ultrasound scanning may be aspirated. Small cysts are left alone. If the mass is palpable and ultrasound has been unhelpful, scintimammography followed by an FNA core biopsy is indicated. If this is cystic then no follow-up is required.

False negative mammograms may occur, e.g. where the pattern of the density is not characteristically spiculated or if calcification within the tumour is absent. However, they are palpable and should be suitable to fine needle aspiration biopsy (FNAB) allowing a correct diagnosis to be made. However, FNAB may be inaccurate because of the poor location of the biopsy or insufficient tissue extracted. Therefore, in patients with multiple suspect areas which appear negative on mammography, scintimammography can guide the FNAB to the most likely area for biopsy.

For secondary or recurrent breast cancers

The X-ray mammogram is usually abnormal in these patients due to scarring from previous surgery or radiotherapy. The ability of ^{99m}Tc sestamibi scintimammography to identify recurrent cancer despite these architectural abnormalities makes it ideal in these patients. This is especially important if the suspected cancer is at the site of a previous operation. In addition, tumour in regional lymph nodes and other tissues, e.g. in the chest wall, can be seen on the scintimammography but not on mammography. Serial imaging may also help to plan treatment and evaluate the therapeutic response.

KEY POINTS
- Scintimammography can be included in the diagnostic and treatment algorithms for breast cancer providing useful additional information for guiding further tests and treatments
- Scintimammography is useful in the evaluation of both primary and recurrent breast cancer

Chapter Seven

The future development of scintimammography

The future development of scintimammography

Scintimammography is becoming established as a diagnostic and management decision-making tool in breast cancer. Meanwhile, other roles for ^{99m}Tc sestamibi scintimammography are emerging. Research is evaluating scintimammography in assessing response to chemotherapy and in planning initial therapy. New high resolution sensitive detectors are being investigated in the hope of identifying tumours of 4-5mm diameter.

[99m]Tc sestamibi scintimammography in assessing a patient's response to chemotherapy

The active mechanism believed to expel ^{99m}Tc sestamibi from cancer cells may prove useful in determining the response of a tumour to chemotherapy and needs to be determined in clinical studies.[1] Resistance to chemotherapy may result in a reduced uptake of ^{99m}Tc sestamibi as it is more quickly expelled from the cell. However, there is insufficient data on this subject at present to determine whether a reduced uptake is a result of the development of resistance or as a direct result of tumour shrinkage. (Figure 1)

There may be a direct temporary reduction in ^{99m}Tc sestamibi uptake in the few months following chemotherapy which is independent of clinical response. Varrela *et al* showed that 19 out of 29 patients had a decrease in ^{99m}Tc sestamibi uptake after chemotherapy.[2] Evidence for a more specific link comes from Naples[3] where a good correlation was seen between the expression of Pgp within the cell and the rate of efflux of ^{99m}Tc sestamibi. (Figure 2) Biopsy samples taken after surgery were stained for Pgp. Again a good correlation occurred between the degree of staining for Pgp and efflux of the ^{99m}Tc sestamibi. The results are still experimental and how this would correlate to predicting clinical response is unclear at present, although the research is promising.

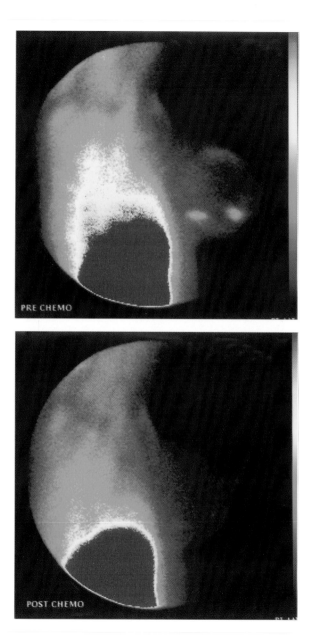

Figure 1   *Pre- and post-chemotherapy treatment images illustrating the reduced activity uptake in the tumour after treatment*

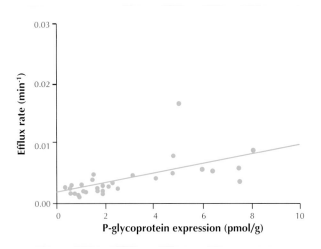

Figure 2   *Correlation between efflux rate of ⁹⁹ᵐTc sestamibi and P-glycoprotein expression in 30 breast carcinomas (Pearson's coefficient of correlation r=0.62 p<0.001)³*

Scintimammography as a management tool for planning therapy

Scintimammography is expected to have a role in the planning of therapy for patients with primary breast cancer, allowing treatments to be tailored for specific patients. The full extent of disease can be seen with scintimammography so that the most effective surgery can be planned from the outset. It may be possible to predict which patients will not respond to primary chemotherapy. Thus, expensive treatment could then be saved for those who would have the best clinical response.

Improving detectors

The modern gamma camera has at best a resolution of 7-10mm and can not be improved in its present form. Solid state detectors are being developed in Southern California which have a small field of view, e.g. 15 x 15cm. This will limit their utility in most nuclear medicine imaging but is an advantage in breast imaging as it will allow the camera to get closer to the breast. At present, the resolution of such a system is similar to an Anger gamma camera but further work should reduce this to a 5mm resolution. This would improve the sensitivity of the system similar to that seen with MRI.

A system is also being developed to permit stereotactic localisation biopsy of an impalpable scintimammographic abnormality not seen on X-ray mammography. The breast is held in a special table with radioactive markers at 1cm distant, in three planes. A fine wire is passed into the tumour until the radioactive tip coincides with the abnormality seen on the scintimammogram in all three planes. The wire is fixed and the patient goes to the operating theatre. The area of the breast around the tip of the wire is removed, scanned and sent for histological examination.

Conclusions

Scintimammography is a nuclear medicine technique which is providing valuable, additional information to that obtained by traditional anatomical screening and assessment. With care, ^{99m}Tc sestamibi scintimammography can provide accurate and important information in women where X-ray mammography is difficult, equivocal or non-diagnostic. This will help the surgeon, physician and oncologist achieve a more accurate diagnosis and plan treatment strategies more efficiently. Surgery and biopsy can be more precise and women need only undergo the minimum necessary surgical intervention.

Scintimammography should not replace mammography or ultrasonography. Rather ^{99m}Tc sestamibi scintimammography should be used to provide complementary information to improve diagnosis and evaluation of breast cancer. It provides answers to questions raised by mammography and helps to reduce the stress and anxiety which patients feel when undergoing tests for breast cancer by providing an increased certainty of diagnosis.

The future of scintimammography seems certain to include a wider role in diagnosis as well as in the planning and evaluation of treatment of breast cancer. More research is needed to assess its clinical value such as its role in the imaging of young women with a high risk for breast cancer.

KEY POINTS

- Scintimammography is a valuable tool in the diagnosis and evaluation of breast cancer
- It may also have an important role in assessing the development of resistance to chemotherapy in women with breast cancer
- Scintimammography may also prove useful in determining appropriate treatments for patients with breast cancer

Chapter One - Introduction

1. Miller AB. Breast cancer epidemiology, etiology, and prevention. In: Harris JR, Hellman S, Hendersen IC. Kinne DW eds. *Breast Diseases*. JB Lippincott Co. Philadelphia 1987; 87-102.
2. From Parkin DM *et al*. Cancer incidence in five continents. [SEER - Surveillance, Epidemiology and End Results program]. Volume VI. Lyon: IARC Scientific Publications n. 120, 1992.
3. Helzlsouer KJ. Epidemiology, prevention, and early detection of breast cancer. *Curr Opin Oncol* 1994; **6**: 541-548.
4. Schouten LJ *et al*. Cancer incidence: life table risk versus cumulative risk. *J Epidemiol Community Health* 1994; **48**: 596-600.
5. Broeders MJM, Verbeek ALM. Breast cancer epidemiology and risk factors. *QJ Nucl Med* 1997; **41**: 179-188.
6. Sondik RJ. Breast cancer trends, incidence, mortality and survival. *Cancer* 1994; **74**: 995-999.
7. Seltzer MH. The significance of breast complaints as correlated with age and breast cancer. *Am Surg* 1992; **58**: 413-417.
8. Anderson I. Mammographic screening and mortality from breast cancer: the Malmo mammographic screening trial. *Br J Med* 1988; **297**: 943-948.
9. Frisell J *et al*. Randomized study of mammography screening - preliminary report on mortality in the Stockholm trial. *Breast Cancer Res Treat* 1991; **18**: 49-56.
10. Miller AB *et al*. The Canadian National Breast Screening Study. *Can Med Associ J* 1992; **147**: 1459-88.
11. Shapiro S *et al*. Current results of the breast cancer screening randomized trial: The Health Insurance Plan (HIP) of Greater New York Study. In: Day NE, Miller AL eds. Screening for Breast Cancer, Hans Huber, Toronto: 1988; 3-15.
12. Waxman AD. The role of ^{99m}Tc methoxyisobutylisonitrile in imaging breast cancer. *Seminars in Nuclear Medicine* 1997; **27**: 40-54.

Chapter Two - The diagnosis of breast cancer

1. Kelsey JL. Gammon MD. The epidemiology of breast cancer. *Cancer* 1991; **41**: 146-165.
2. Maublant JC *et al*. Hexakis (2-methoxyisobutyl-isonitrile) technetium -99m and thallium-201 chloride: Uptake and release in cultured myocardial cells. *J Nucl Med* 1988; **29**: 48-53.
3. Fletcher SW *et al*. Report of the International Workshop on Screening of Breast Cancer. *J National Cancer Inst* 1993; **85**: 1644-1656.
4. Waxman AD. The role of ^{99m}Tc methoxyisobutylisonitrile in imaging breast cancer. *Seminars in Nuclear Medicine* 1997; **27**: 40-54.
5. Madjar H *et al*. Value of high resolution sonography in breast cancer screening. *Ultraschall Med* 1994; **15**: 20-23.
6. Kopans DB. What is a useful adjunct to mammography? *Radiology* 1986; **161**: 560-561.

7. Teubner J. Echomammography: technique and results. In: Friedrick M, Sickles EA, eds. Radiological diagnosis of breast diseases. Berlin, Heidelberg, New York: Springer, 1997; 291-298.
8. Orel S *et al*. High-resolution MR imaging of the breast: Clinical context. *Radiographics* 1996; **16** (6): 1385-1401.
9. Mussarakis S *et al*. Dynamic MR imaging of the breast combined with analysis of contrast agent kinetics in the differentiation of primary breast tumours. *Clinical Radiology* 1997; **52**: 516-526.
10. Oellinger H *et al*. Gd-TDTPA enhanced MRI of the breast: the most sensitive method for detecting multicentric carcinomas in female breast? *Eur Radiol* 1993; **2**: 223-224.
11. Harms SE *et al*. MR imaging of the breast with rotating delivery of excitation of resonance: Clinical experience with pathological correlation. *Radiology* 1993; **187**: 493-501.
12. Nguyen K *et al*. Comparison of Tc-99m methoxyisobutylisonitrile and MRI in breast malignancy: The significance of concordant and discordant findings. *J Nucl ed* 1996; **37**: 75P (abstract).
13. Harms SE *et al*. Fat-suppressed three dimensional MR imaging of the breast. *Radiographics* 1993; **13**: 247-267.
14. The Royal College of Radiologists. Contrast enhanced MR imaging. *Clinical Radiology* 1996; **51**: 235-244.
15. Crowe JP *et al*. Positron emission tomography and breast masses: Comparison with clinical, mammographic and pathological finding. *Ann Surg Oncol* 1994; **1**: 1132-1140.
16. Tse NY *et al*. The application of positron emission tomographic imaging with fluorodeoxyglucose to the evaluation of breast disease. *Annals of Surgery* 1992; **216**: 27-34.
17. Adler LP *et al*. Evaluation of breast masses and axillary lymph nodes with [F-18] 2-deoxy-2-fluoro-D-glucose PET. *Radiology* 1993; **187**: 743-750.
18. Bombardieri E. Nuclear medicine techniques for the study of breast cancer. *Eur J Nucl Med* 1997; **24**: 809-824.
19. Buscombe J *et al*. Scintigraphic imaging of breast cancer: A review. *Nuclear Medicine Communications* 1997; **18**: 698-709.

Chapter Three - The rationale for scintimammography

1. Bombardieri E. Nuclear medicine techniques for the study of breast cancer. *Eur J Nucl Med* 1997; **24**: 809-824.
2. Cox PH *et al*. Thallium 201 chloride uptake in tumours, a possible complication in heart scintigraphy. *Br J Radiol* 1976; **49**: 767-768.
3. Khalkhali I *et al*. Prone scintimammography in patients with suspicion of carcinoma of the breast. *J Am Coll Surg* 1994; **178**: 491-497.
4. Khalkhali I *et al*. Scintimammography: the new role of technetium-99m sestamibi imaging for the diagnosis of breast carcinoma. *Q J Nucl Med* 1997; **41**: 231-238.
5. Maublant JC *et al*. Hexakis (2-methoxyisobutyl-isonitrile) technetium-99m and thallium-201 chloride: Uptake and release in cultured myocardial cells. *J Nucl Med* 1988; **29**: 48-53.

6. Buscombe J et al. Scintigraphic imaging of breast cancer: A review. *Nuclear Medicine Communications* 1997; **18**: 698-709.
7. Waxman AD. The role of ^{99m}Tc methoxyisobutylisonitrile in imaging breast cancer. *Seminars in Nuclear Medicine* 1997; **27**: 40-54.
8. Goldstein et al. Expression of a multi-drug resistance gene in human cancers. *J Natl Cancer Inst* 1989; **81**: 116-120.
9. Piwnica-Worms D et al. Noncardiac applications of hexakis (alkylisonitrile) technetium-99 complexes. *J Nucl Med* 1990; **31**: 1166-1167.
10. Palmedo H et al. Scintimammography with technetium-99m methoxyisobutylisonitrile: comparison with mammography and magnetic resonance imaging. *Eur J Nuc Med* 1996; **23**: 940-946.
11. Burak et al. Evaluation of palpable breast masses with Tc99m-MIBI: a comparative study with mammography and ultrasonography. *Nucl Med Comm* 1994; **15**: 604-612.
12. Kao et al. The use of technetium-99m methoxyisobutyl-isonitrile breast scintigraphy to evaluate palpable breast masses. *Eur J Nucl Med* 1994; **21**: 432-436.
13. Khalkhali I et al. Prone scintimammography in patients with suspicion of carcinoma of the breast. *J Am Coll Surg* 1994; **178**: 491-497.
14. Lu et al. Tc 99m sestamibi mammoscintigraphy of breast masses: Early and delayed imaging. *Nucl Med Comm* 1995; **16**: 150-156.
15. Vicioso et al. Breast scintigraphy with technetium Tc 99m sestamibi in the evaluation of tumor pathology. *Preliminary Results Rev Esp Med Nucl* 1994; **13** (6): 269-274.
16. Piccolo S et al. Scintimammography with 99mTc-MDP in the detection of early breast cancer. *Q J Nucl Med* 1997; **41**: 225-230.

Chapter Four - The clinical role of scintimammography

1. Jackson VP et al. Imaging of the radiographically dense breast. *Radiology* 1993; **188**: 297-301.
2. Saphner T et al. Annual hazard rates of recurrence for breast cancer after primary therapy. *J Clin Oncol* 1996; **14**: 2738-2746.
3. Villanueve-Meyer S et al. Impact of breast density on the diagnostic accuracy of ^{99m}Tc sestamibi breast imaging in the detection of breast cancer. *J Nucl Med* 1996; **37** (5): 74.
4. Krag K et al. Surgical resection and radio-localization of the sentinel lymph node in breast cancer using gamma probe. *Surg Oncol* 1993; **2**: 335-340.
5. National Institute for Health Consensus Conference. Treatment of early stage breast cancer. *JAMA* 1991; **265**: 391-395.

Chapter Five - Performing high quality scintimammography with ^{99m}Tc sestamibi

1. Piwnica-Worms D *et al.* Noncardiac applications of hexakis (alkylisonitrile) technetium-99 complexes. *J Nucl Med* 1990; **31**: 1166-1167.
2. Khalkhali I *et al.* Prone scintimammography in patients with suspicion of carcinoma of the breast. *J Am Coll Surg* 1994; **178**: 491-497.

Chapter Six - Incorporating scintimammography into the diagnosis and management of breast cancer

1. Oellinger H *et al.* Gd-DTPA enhanced MRI of the breast: the most sensitive method for detecting multicentric carcinomas in female breast? *Eur Radiol* 1993; **2**: 223-226.
2. Harms SE *et al.* MR imaging of the breast with rotating delivery of excitation of resonance: Clinical experience with pathological correlation. *Radiology* 1993; **187**: 493-501.
3. Nguyen K *et al.* Comparison of Tc-99m methoxyisobutylisonitrile (MIBI) and MRI in breast malignancy: The significance of concordant and discordant findings. *J Nucl ed* 1996; **37**: 75P (abstract).

Chapter Seven - The future development of scintimammography

1. Piwnica-Worms D *et al.* Noncardiac applications of hexakis (alkylisonitrile) technetium-99 complexes. *J Nucl Med* 1990; **31**: 1166-1167.
2. Varrela P *et al.* Tc 99m MIBI scintimammography for monitoring tumour response in patients with advanced breast cancer. *J Nucl Med* 1995; **36** (suppl 5): 193 (abstract 869).
3. Del Vecchio *et al. In vivo* detection of mulitdrug resistant (MDR1) phenotype by technetium-99m sestamibi scan in untreated breast cancer patients. *Euro J Nuc Med* 1997; **24**: 150-159.

References